COLPOSCOPY
IN CLINICAL PRACTICE

COLPOSCOPY
IN CLINICAL PRACTICE

Louis Burke, M.D.
Assistant Director
Department of Obstetrics and Gynecology
Chief, Department of Clinical Obstetrics
and Colposcopy Clinic
Beth Israel Hospital
Boston, Massachusetts

Assistant Professor
of Obstetrics and Gynecology
Harvard Medical School
Boston, Massachusetts

Barbara E. Mathews, M.D.
Department of Obstetrics and Gynecology
Beth Israel Hospital
Boston, Massachusetts

Instructor in Obstetrics and Gynecology
Harvard Medical School
Boston, Massachusetts

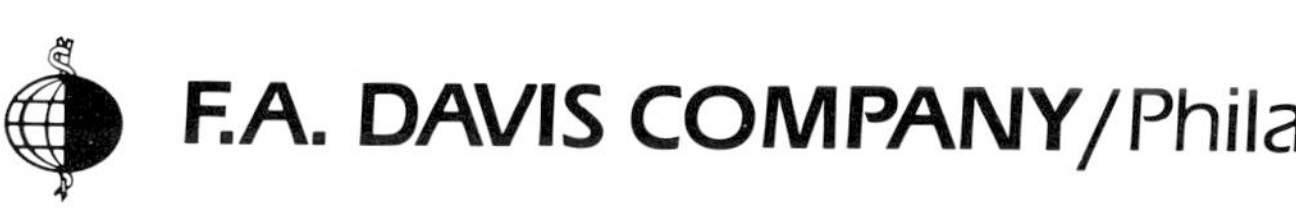
F.A. DAVIS COMPANY/Philadelphia

Printed in the United States of America

Library of Congress Cataloging in Publication Data

Burke, Louis.
Colposcopy in clinical practice.

Bibliography: p.
Includes index. 1. Colposcopy. I. Mathews, Barbara E., joint author. II. Title. [DNLM: 1. Colposcopy. WP250 B959c]
RG107.5.C6B87 618.1'4'0754 77-21063
ISBN 0-8036-1425-X

This book is dedicated with much gratitude and affection by
Louis Burke to his wife, Dorothy
and
Barbara Matthews to her parents,
Dr. and Mrs. J. Chesley Matthews.

FOREWORD

Colposcopy has only recently approached its proper place as an important ancillary aid in the practice of gynecology in this country. Despite its late rebirth and popularization here, colposcopy has been recognized as a valuable clinical tool abroad for nearly half a century, since shortly after it was first introduced by Hinselmann in 1925. Our collective reluctance to pursue this modality with comparable enthusiasm here may have been based on a prevalent misinterpretation of its role. It has long been denigrated—quite inappropriately—because it was considered an unacceptable competitor of cytologic methods as a means of screening large populations for gynecologic cancer. Clearly, colposcopy cannot be considered a substitute for cytology in this regard. It neither competes with nor duplicates cytology; but it can and does serve a most critical function in complementing the use of cytology, serving to help study those patients designated by the cytologic screening process as potentially at risk, and focusing upon those specific sites warranting biopsy for histologic examination. Indeed, colposcopy stands between cytology and histology—that is, between population screening and definitive tissue diagnosis.

This volume serves not only as a handy manual and practical technical guide but also as a survey reference resource and atlas. It provides lucid and succinct information for rapid assimilation by the practicing physician. The clarity of both the prose and the illustrative material is admirable. The excellent colpophotography is a credit to the authors and to the publisher. The reader should find this book useful as a simplified basic teaching course for the novice; alternatively, it will prove valuable as a helpful review for those who already have some clinical experience with this important technological advance. It can be highly recommended for both leisurely reading and intensive study.

Emanuel A. Friedman, M.D., Sc.D.
Professor of Obstetrics and Gynecology
Harvard Medical School

PREFACE

The cervix and vagina first became accessible for direct inspection as a result of the invention of the vaginal speculum by Récamier in 1818. As a consequence, investigators were able to turn their attention to elucidating the natural history of cervical cancer.

By the turn of the century, gynecologists shifted their focus of interest from the gross and histologic appearance of advanced disease to the less well defined subject of preclinical carcinoma of the cervix. Hinselmann in 1925 made a most significant contribution in this regard. He conjectured that the primary focus of cervical cancer may be a minute ulceration or nodule which could be appreciated only with low power magnification and high intensity illumination. He devised the colposcope for inspection of the cervix with sharply focused light and binocular optical magnification, thus pioneering a new field of clinical investigation, colposcopy.

Hinselmann's method of cervical evaluation was widely accepted and enthusiastically promoted throughout Europe. Colposcopy became a part of every routine gynecologic examination and was utilized as the primary method of cervical cancer screening and detection. The meticulous examination of thousands of patients with the colposcope enabled Hinselmann to define many benign changes on the cervix. With the aid of directed biopsy, he was able to correlate atypical changes with early cancerous or precancerous lesions. He could not find the minute foci of ulceration or nodularity he expected; instead, the colposcope disclosed a variety of epithelial changes corresponding to different benign and malignant histologic patterns. His observations served as the foundation upon which our present day concepts of the origin of cervical cancer were built. Cancer begins not in a focus of static tissue but within a sheet of dynamically changing epithelium.

Until recently, colposcopy was not widely used by gynecologists in the English-speaking countries, with the exception of Australia. Efforts to introduce the technique in the United States began around 1930, but were largely unsuccessful. The delay in its adoption may be attributed to the fact that all the reports of the initial work were published in German. Terminology was based on visual impressions, such as "ground substance," and could not be clearly related to the histology or pathophysiology of tumor growth and development. It was not until 1960 that English reports first placed colposcopy on a logical scientific basis and provided correlation between colposcopic and clinical terminology.

Acceptance of colposcopy into American gynecologic practice was also impeded by the introduction in the 1940s of the Papanicolaou smear for diagnostic exfoliative cytology in screening for carcinoma or dysplasia of the cervix. Cytology and colposcopy were initially construed as competitive rather than as complementary techniques. For detection of cervical cancer, colposcopy proved to be somewhat less reliable than cytology. Moreover, cytology was much more economical, less time consuming, and more easily adapted to mass screening programs. Proper training and special instruments imported from abroad were needed for colposcopy. Additionally, it was difficult to describe complicated visual patterns adequately. Findings were first recorded by hand drawings. The limitation imposed by inaccurate sketches was overcome when improved optics made photography feasible.

The virtues of combining cytology and colposcopy for cervical cancer detection were first recognized by Navratil and Limberg in 1958. In a series of patients with preclinical cervical carcinoma who were examined simultaneously by colposcopy and cytology, Navratil reported detection by cytology or colposcopy alone in approximately 85 percent of cases. Employed together, both methods detected 99 percent of cases. Each method compensated for the deficiencies of the other. More recent studies have corroborated these findings.

Current investigations now support a major role for colposcopy in the vaginal examination of women exposed to diethylstilbestrol in utero. In addition, colposcopy has been used in evaluating vulvar disease.

Colposcopy, especially during the past few years, has come to enjoy growing interest in the United States. This interest has been manifested by the development of teaching aids, instructional and photographic techniques, and American-made equipment. New reference materials have been published along with numerous articles citing the many advantages of the use of colposcopy in the evaluation of gynecologic disease. Many gynecologists have acquired a thorough understanding of the technique and practice of colposcopy. A few of them offer hospital-based consultation and direct seminars so that an ever increasing number of gynecologists can apply this diagnostic tool in their own practices. Our colposcopy course at Harvard is only one of many graduate training sessions given annually in this country, attesting to the interest in this subject among clinical gynecologists. Residents are now being trained in this skill. Many gynecologists are purchasing colposcopes for office use. The requests we have had from local gynecologists for assistance in reviewing techniques and basic principles have in part prompted the publication of this manual.

We have written this general review of colposcopy primarily

for medical students, residents, and practicing gynecologists who wish to become familiar with the field by means of an illustrated text. Our objective is to provide an easily readable account of indications for and technical details of the procedure, along with a discussion of the principles and histologic basis of colposcopy. We have tried to combine a simplified overview of material that is presented in greater depth in reference monographs with the attributes of a technical guide and atlas. Since the concept of colposcopy depends primarily on the appreciation of visual image, illustrations are presented in color to provide accurate and comprehensible representations of clinical material. Our photographs are views of the cervix as it is actually observed and recorded by the clinical gynecologist rather than views obtained with sophisticated equipment and techniques utilized in study and research.

Colposcopy is still a subject of considerable debate. It has its greatest applications (1) in the practical evaluation and precise diagnosis of lesions of the cervix, vagina, and vulva, and (2) in investigational research directed at furthering our understanding of the etiology and pathogenesis of benign and malignant disease in these organs. This manual is concerned solely with the first of these aims.

Colposcopy is a clinical tool. It is not a difficult procedure. It is easily taught and readily learned, but it should be emphasized that, without proper training, serious mistakes can be made and subtle benefits may never be realized.

L.B.
B.E.M.

ACKNOWLEDGMENTS

This manual is the culmination not only of our own labors but also of the efforts of many other industrious and dedicated individuals. We are grateful to the Beth Israel Hospital Out-Patient Department and to many private gynecologists on the staff of the Beth Israel Hospital for providing the patient material photographed herein. Special thanks are extended to Mrs. Paula Sawyer, R.N., for her impeccable assistance during virtually every colposcopic examination.

Our special consideration is given to Miss Patricia L. Allen who devoted her valuable hours and secretarial skills to collating and typing material for this book. We are grateful also to Mrs. Harriet R. Greenfield who provided our medical illustrations.

This book continues to be a reminder to us of the support and instruction provided by many professors. We are especially grateful to Emanuel A. Friedman, M.D., who offered suggestions and encouragement throughout this endeavor.

We appreciate the support, advice, and patience of our publisher, F. A. Davis Company. We thank their President, Mr. Robert H. Craven, and their accomplished medical editor, Mrs. Christine H. Young, for technical assistance.

CONTENTS

1

INSTRUMENTATION

The colposcope serves to evaluate subtle changes in the surface pattern and terminal vascular network of pelvic tissues. In order to provide the required topographic orientation, any colposcope must include the essential components of magnification, high intensity illumination, and stereoscopic viewing. Photographic recording is desirable although not essential.

CONSTRUCTION

All colposcopes consist of a stereoscopic binocular microscope with low magnification, usually 10× to 40×. The instrument is equipped with a centered illuminating device which may be mounted in a variety of ways. The light source most often is an incandescent lamp with a rheostat to alter the light intensity. A remote tungsten halogen lamp may also serve this purpose, with its illumination adjusted by a potentiometer and brought to the instrument through a fiberoptic cable. Fiberoptic lighting tends to be cooler for both the patient and the colposcopist.

The colposcope may be placed on an adjustable stand with a transformer in the base, affixed to the side of an examining table to be swung out, or even attached to the ceiling to be pulled down and centered for the examination of a patient (Figs. 1 to 4). Attachment to the examining table seems preferable for the

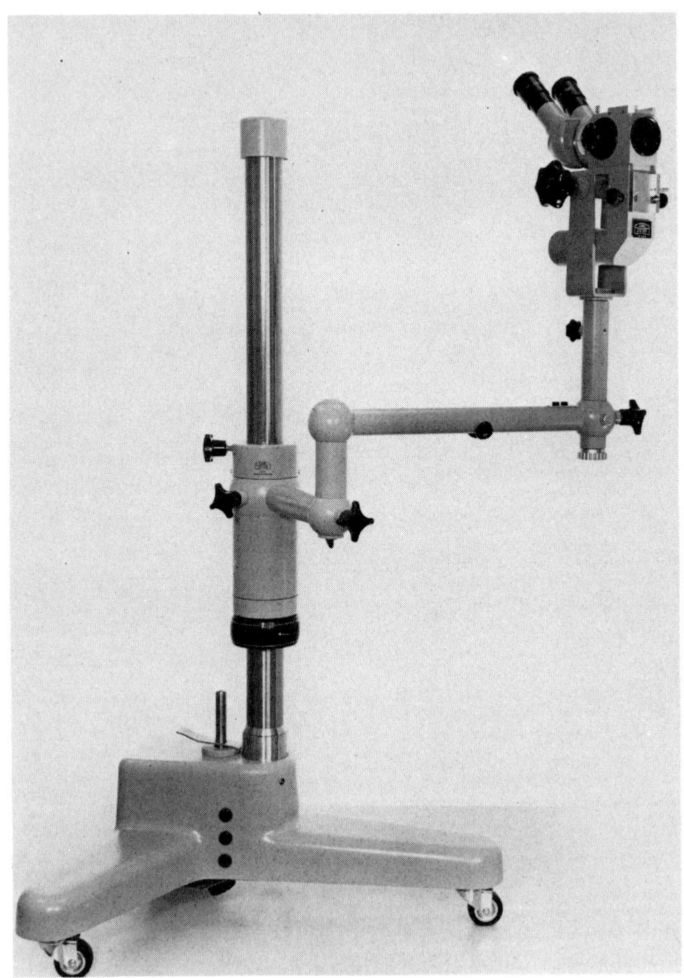

Figure 1. Zeiss colposcope 1 positioned on a system of pivotal arms and attached to a heavy mobile base. (Courtesy Carl Zeiss, Inc., New York.)

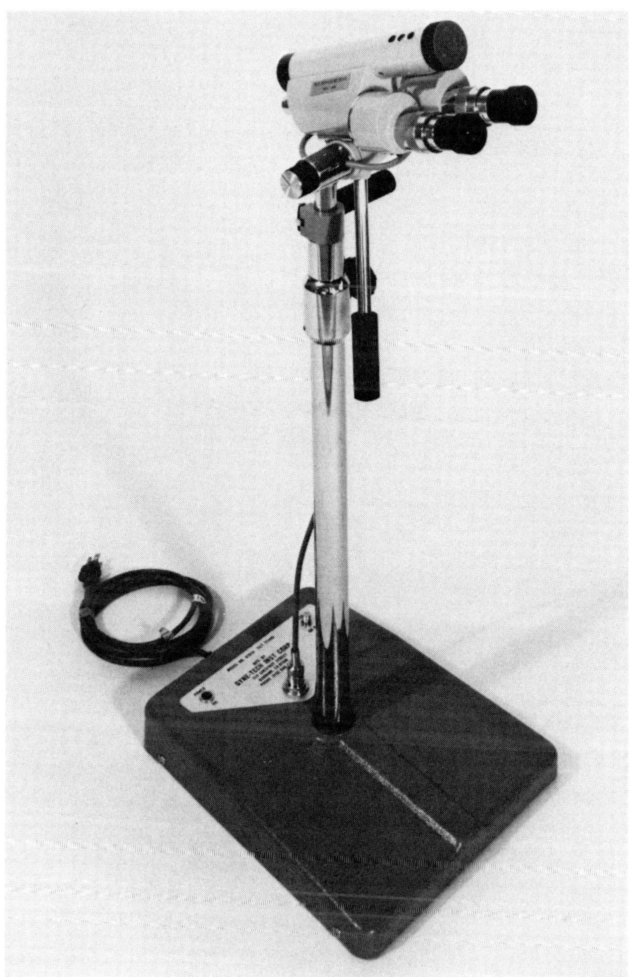

Figure 2. Colposcope on light-weight mobile base. (Courtesy Gyné-Tech Instrument Corporation, Burbank, California.)

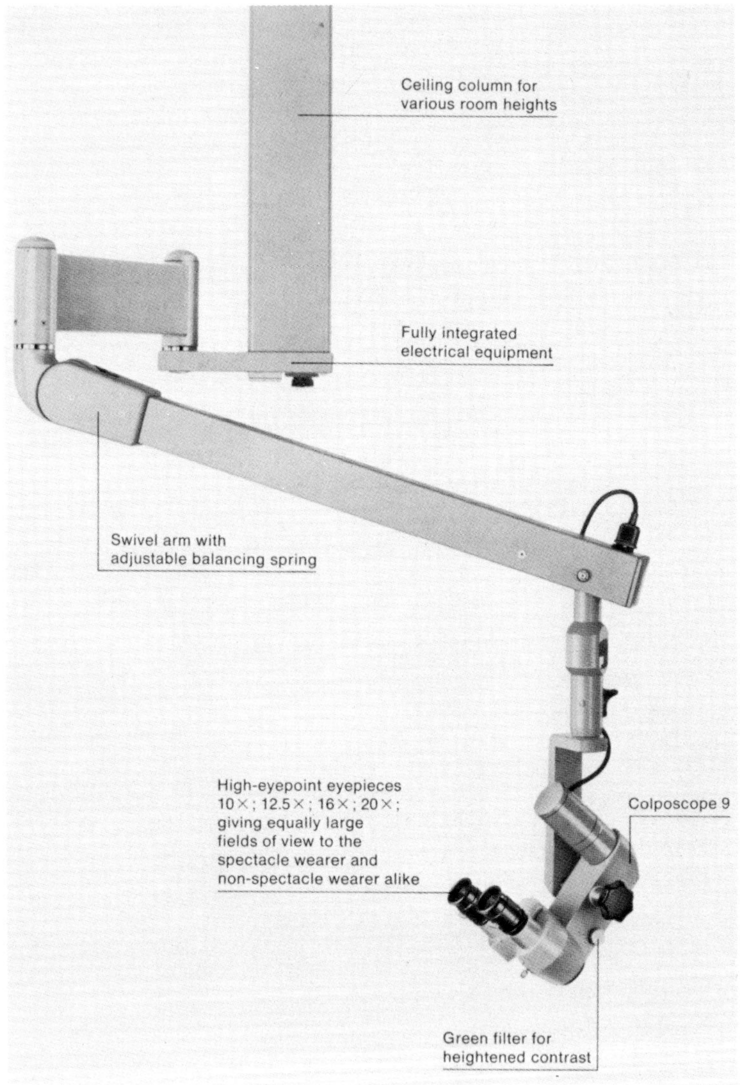

Figure 3. Zeiss colposcope 9 on ceiling-mounted column with swivel arm. (Courtesy Carl Zeiss, Inc., New York.)

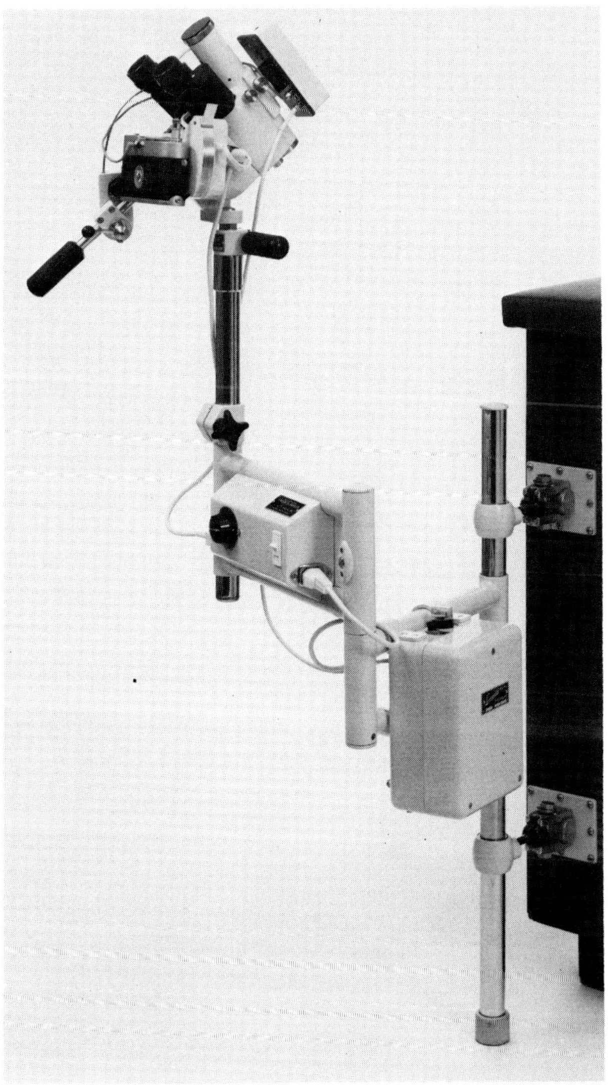

Figure 4. Leisegang colposcope IIIB attached to an examining table by a "Swing-O-Matic" mount. (Courtesy Gynemed, Inc., Palo Alto, Calif.)

gynecologist's private office. However, with this arrangement, one may also wish to purchase a simple mobile stand so that the colposcopic head can be removed from the table and transported by stand for use in an operating room.

OPTICS

There are many colposcopes commercially available in this country, both of foreign and American manufacture. Specifically, these include those marketed by Frigitronics, Applied Fiberoptics, Cryomedics, International Micro-Optics, Toitu, Berkeley Bioengineering, Dynatech, Jena, Zeiss, and Leisegang. The type of instrument purchased should depend somewhat on the character of the work for which it is intended.

By virtue of their optics, colposcopes fall into two general categories, those containing multiple objectives built into a single optical unit (i.e., with several available magnifications, a feature of Toitu, Jena, and Zeiss instruments), and those exhibiting a single objective (i.e., with fixed magnification). In the fixed focus instruments, the magnification can be altered only by changing the eyepieces; these may be obtained in magnifications varying from 5× to 20×.

The optics supplied by the different manufacturers can be tailored to the type of work required. The optics influence the working distance between the instrument and the field of examination. The best focal length for a working colposcope is between 200 and 250 mm. Colposcopes are generally fitted with lenses to provide focal lengths within this range (with the exception of the Berkeley instrument which has a standard focal length of 300 mm). With a working distance of 200 to 250 mm between the objective lens and the field of examination, the colposcope does not enter the vagina. Punch biopsies, scrapings, and treatments can be carried out under the visual guidance provided by the colposcope. One may find some difficulty and awkwardness at this focal length if one uses biopsy instruments that are longer than 20 to 25 cm. Consequently, instruments such as curettes, endocervical specula, and biopsy forceps should, where possible, be limited to the shorter 15 cm length rather than the 25 cm length in common use. A focal length of 300 mm is more appropriate when long instruments are being used. A short focal length of 100 to 200 mm is often valuable for obtaining photographic records for teaching or research purposes.

A separate handle is provided on all instruments for free movement of the focusing element. Care should always be taken to align the colposcope so that the light beam strikes the observed tissue at right angles. With a focal length of 200 to 250 mm and 10× magnification, the diameter of a visualized field ranges in different colposcopes from 20 to 23 mm. This width of exposure permits one to observe and contrast atypical areas with adjacent normal tissue. It is important to keep in mind that lengthening the focal length at any given magnification will increase the diameter of the exposed field.

ACCESSORIES

The binocular eyepieces of all instruments may have independent focusing elements and are adjustable for individual intraocular distance. They may be fitted with special rubber cups for eyeglass wearers. The angle of the eyepieces, relative to the long axis of the instrument, is also variable and should be modified for comfort and ease of viewing. In many colposcopes, a built-in micrometer permits one to measure the size of involved areas.

Most instruments are provided with a green filter for purposes of interposition between the light source and the area being viewed. The green filter absorbs red from the color spectrum, permitting blood vessels to stand out in detail as black objects. Since it increases contrast and accentuates vascular morphology, the green filter is a mandatory accessory.

BASIC COLPOSCOPES

The photographs printed in this publication were obtained with the use of two types of colposcope, the Zeiss and the Leisegang

Series IIIB. The characteristics of these instruments will be detailed, recognizing that other commercial colposcopes display essentially the same technical features, with slight modifications in style and design as well as in magnification, light intensity, and type of green filter.

The Zeiss colposcope is comprised of a modified operating microscope positioned on a system of pivoting arms, mounted on a heavy mobile base. Construction allows for universal movement and easy manipulation. The optical head, which contains a 6 volt, 30 watt lamp, provides high intensity illumination along the optical pathway. By means of a 3-way switch, the voltage can be increased to brighten the illumination and spotlight any particular area. The Zeiss colposcope provides multiple magnifications. Magnification is changed simply by

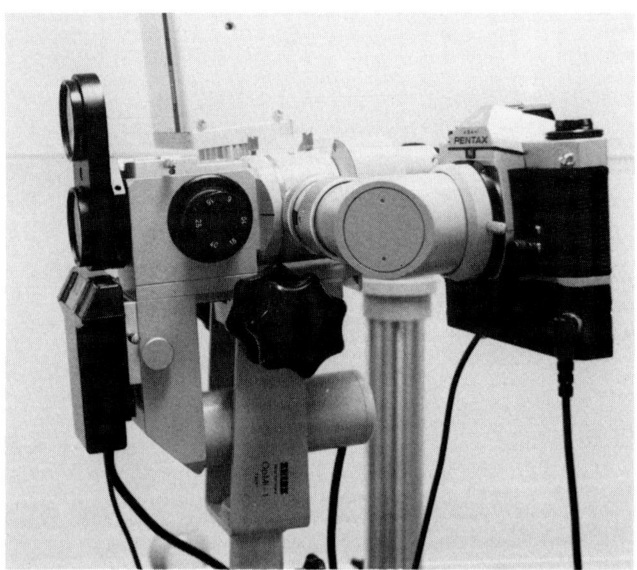

Figure 5. Head of Zeiss colposcope 1 showing Galilean magnification changer. (Courtesy Carl Zeiss, Inc., New York.)

turning a knob with varied settings (designated 6, 10, 16, 25, and 40) without the need for refocusing (Fig. 5). It is important to recognize that the number of the setting does not represent the degree of magnification. At any given setting, magnification is altered by the objective lens and the strength of the oculars (Table 1).

Table 1. Magnification Table. Colposcopic field magnifications related to focal length of objective lens, ocular strength, and Galilean changer setting (for Zeiss colposcope). (Courtesy Carl Zeiss, Inc., New York.)

Working Distance		*Eyepieces*	*Total magnifications with settings:*				
Inch	*mm*		*6*	*10*	*16*	*25*	*40*
		10 ×	2.5×	4 ×	6 ×	10 ×	16 ×
8	200	12.5×	3 ×	5 ×	8 ×	12.5×	20 ×
		16 ×	4 ×	6 ×	10 ×	16 ×	25 ×
		20 ×	5 ×	8 ×	12.5×	20 ×	32 ×
		10 ×	2.2×	3.5×	5.5×	9 ×	14 ×
9	225	12.5×	2.8×	4.5×	7 ×	11.5×	18 ×
		16 ×	3.5×	5.5×	9 ×	14.5×	23 ×
		20 ×	4.5×	7 ×	11 ×	18 ×	28 ×
		10 ×	2 ×	3 ×	5 ×	8 ×	13 ×
10	250	12.5×	2.5×	4 ×	6 ×	10 ×	16 ×
		16 ×	3 ×	5 ×	8 ×	13 ×	20 ×
		20 ×	4 ×	6 ×	10 ×	16 ×	25 ×
		10 ×	1.8×	2.5×	4.5×	7 ×	11.5×
11	275	12.5×	2.3×	3.5×	5.5×	9 ×	15 ×
		16 ×	3 ×	4.5×	7 ×	12 ×	19 ×
		20 ×	3.5×	5 ×	9 ×	15 ×	23 ×
		10 ×	1.5×	2 ×	4 ×	6 ×	10.5×
12	300	12.5×	2 ×	3 ×	5 ×	8 ×	14 ×
		16 ×	2.5×	4 ×	6 ×	11 ×	18 ×
		20 ×	3 ×	4.5×	8 ×	13 ×	19 ×

Valid for straight and inclined binocular tube f = 125 mm

For routine examination, magnification of 10× to 16× is quite satisfactory. When examination of the entire vagina is necessary, as in vaginal adenosis, the lower powers of 5× to 10× offer the advantage of ease of rapid screening. For detailed inspection of the vascular pattern, the magnification should not be less than 13.5×. Magnifications of 20× to 40× may be needed at times for

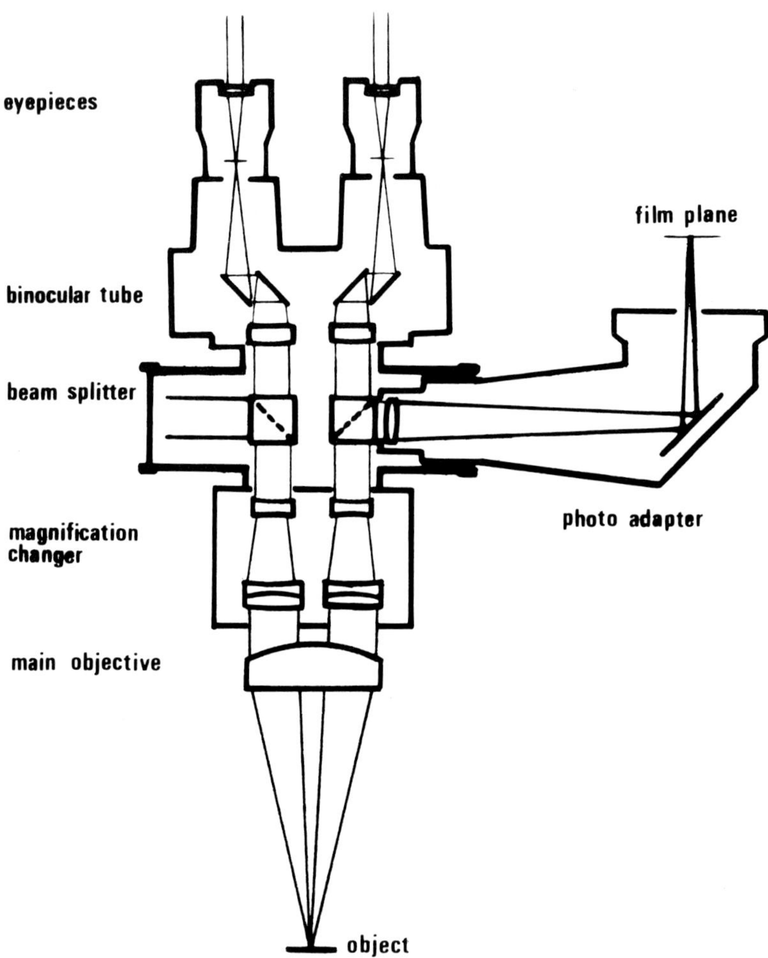

Figure 6. Diagram of optical pathway of Zeiss colposcope demonstrating magnification changer, beam splitter, and photo adapter.

detailed evaluation of abnormal vasculature. However, the benefits of enhanced magnification tend to be outweighed by a decrease in the field of vision, decrease in depth of focus, and loss of architectural orientation.

A photographic unit with a separate optical pathway may be attached to the optical head of the Zeiss colposcope (Fig. 6). The photographic element is focused with the plane of the viewing optics. In general, the Zeiss colposcope is most useful for hospital-based practice and for individuals engaged in investigative research.

The Leisegang colposcope differs in some respects from the Zeiss instrument. Only two magnifications are available—13.5× and 50× (most colposcopes are equipped with the 13.5× objective only). The focused light source is slightly inclined away from the viewing optical pathway. The photographic unit, unlike that of most other colposcopes, is adapted to produce stereoscopic transparencies for use in a special viewer, and is integral with the whole unit. The entire unit may be mounted on a frame for attachment to an examining table. Alternatively, it can be attached to a single pivotal extention arm of a mobile adjustable stand or placed on top of such a stand. Leisegang and other manufacturers offer portable, lightweight, inexpensive colposcopes for the gynecologist for whom cost, maneuverability, and storage space are major considerations.

2

TECHNIQUE

Colposcopy is a relatively simple procedure. It requires familiarity with only a few pieces of equipment. It involves a systematic approach to inspecting tissue, facility in obtaining biopsy specimens, and precise recording of data.

EQUIPMENT

Examination Table

Good colposcopic technique demands correct positioning of patient and instrument for the examination. The patient must assume the dorsal lithotomy position. She will need to maintain this position for a variable length of time, frequently for as long as 30 minutes when biopsies are taken. The examination table, then, should offer both maximal patient comfort and ease of inspection. Tables equipped with an automatic foot control for adjusting height are often helpful (Fig. 7). Special knee and calf supports for the patient are also useful. However, the usual stationary gynecologic tables with conventional stirrups are entirely acceptable for colposcopic examination. Such tables may need to be elevated as much as two inches on wooden blocks in order to perform colposcopic examinations without neck or back strain. The colposcope, whether attached to the examining table

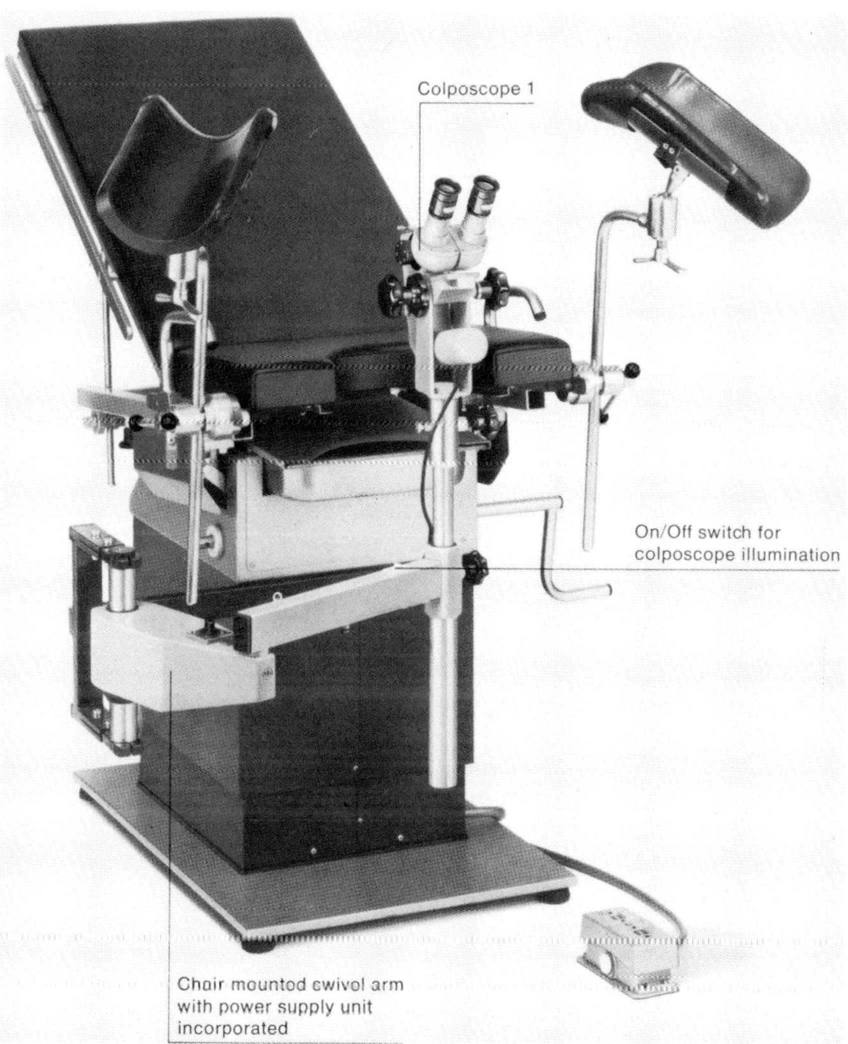

Figure 7. Zeiss colposcope 1 attached to table equipped with automatic controls. (Courtesy Carl Zeiss, Inc., New York.)

or mounted on a free-standing mobile base, is best placed to the left of the examiner in order to provide ample room for those procedures most often performed with the right hand. Accordingly, left-handed physicians should locate their colposcopes on the right. In either case, the colposcope, positioned on a system of pivotal arms, can be expediently centered for the examination. Some colposcopes are fastened to the top of a pole which is attached to a flat stand. Such stands are often somewhat unsteady, and the colposcopist frequently must place his feet on the base of the stand to ensure sturdiness.

Specula

A self-retaining bivalve speculum is needed for adequate visualization of the cervix and vagina. A variety of sizes should be available. The Graves speculum is the type most commonly employed. A speculum longer than 10 cm is seldom required; if used, it may be ejected from the vagina as a result of its unevenly distributed weight. The Pederson and virginal specula are useful for the examination of sexually inactive women. These specula are particularly convenient for evaluating adolescents who were exposed in utero to diethylstilbestrol. Since reflective highlights from conventional stainless steel instruments will distort colpophotographs, it is recommended that these specula be purchased in matte variety stainless steel or with Teflon coating.

The equipment required for colposcopic examination is shown in Figure 8.

THE EXAMINATION

Colposcopic examination may be accomplished by the successful completion of the following three steps:

1. Inspection of the unprepared cervix and vagina, and, when indicated, the vulva.
2. Inspection through the green filter.
3. Inspection following application of acetic acid 3 percent solution.

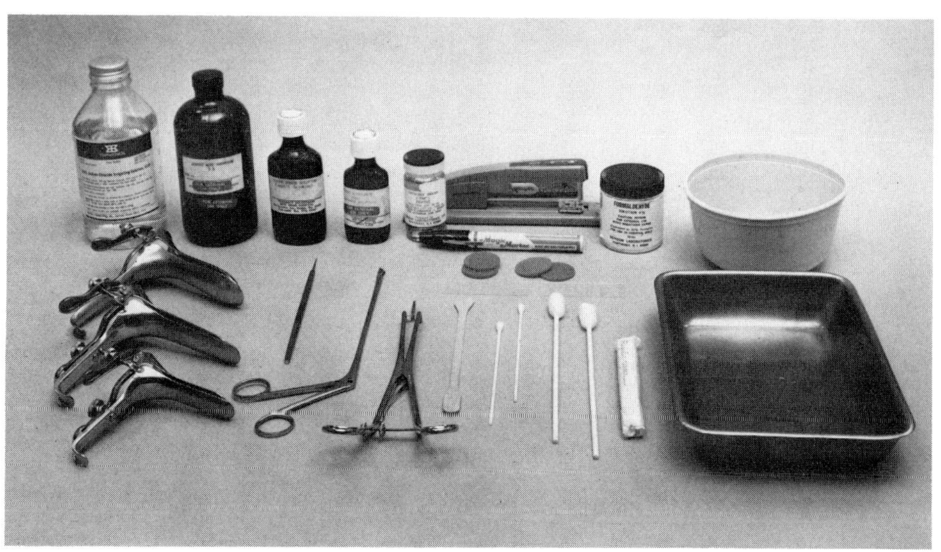

Figure 8. Equipment required for colposcopic examination: Front row (l to r): specula (Graves, Pedersen, virginal), iris hook, Younge-Kevorkian biopsy forceps, Kogan-Martin endocervical speculum, Ayres cervical spatula, cotton-tipped applicators, "Scopettes," tampon, and basin for "Cidex" sterilizing solution. Rear row (l to r): Normal saline, 3% acetic acid, Lugol's iodine solution, Monsel's solution, cytology fixative, material for submitting biopsy specimens (styrofoam circles, Magic Marker, stapler, formalin fixative), and basin for sterile water.

At all times throughout the colposcopic examination, the examiner should look for characteristics of and alterations in epithelial color and opacity, surface contour, clarity of demarcation of tissue patterns, vascular configuration, and intercapillary distance.

Unprepared Tissue

A warm vaginal speculum without lubricant should be introduced slowly into the vagina; the blades of the speculum must be partially separated soon after entry into the vagina to avoid traumatizing the cervix as it is exposed. If necessary, a Papanicolaou smear can be taken concurrently with the colposcopic examination; however, this procedure may initiate bleeding and obliterate features of colposcopic interest. In general, cytologic smears are best taken from the cervix and from the endocervical canal at a separate examination prior to colposcopy.

The vaginal speculum should be held by one hand and manipulated to place the cervix at right angles to the incident light. The other hand should direct the colposcope toward the cervix until focal length is obtained for optimal resolution. Mucus may be removed gently from the cervix with either a dry gauze or one soaked in normal saline. The latter tends to produce less contact bleeding.

The vagina and cervix should be inspected through the colposcope using initially 5× to 16× magnification. For this examination, the cervical and vaginal surfaces should be moistened with normal saline; a dry epithelial surface is not transparent and gives a poor view of vascular patterns.

The purpose of the colposcopic examination of saline-washed tissue is to delineate gross lesions and observe vascular detail. The unprepared epithelium provides no useful information regarding tissue properties such as color or opacity.

Green Filter

Use of the green filter provides the best colposcopic impression of vascular patterns. The green filter absorbs red from the color spectrum; this causes blood vessels to stand out as black structures against a background of white or translucent epithelium.

Acetic Acid

Acetic acid 3 percent solution in water was used first by Hinselmann in 1925. It offers the sharpest contrast between foci of normal and abnormal tissue. For reasons which remain obscure, acetic acid solution shrinks blood vessels, dissolves mucus, and causes individual cells to swell. Transparency of epithelium is greatly reduced and the grape-like structure of columnar tissue enhanced. A change in atypical forms of epithelium occurs. Dysplastic and neoplastic epithelia take on a well demarcated whitish hue. Such epithelia, prior to application of acetic acid, show no distinction in color from normal tissue. A 3 percent solution of acetic acid is generally used for colposcopic examination; 2, 4 percent, or 5 percent dilutions of acetic acid are also acceptable, although less preferable. The weaker dilution re-

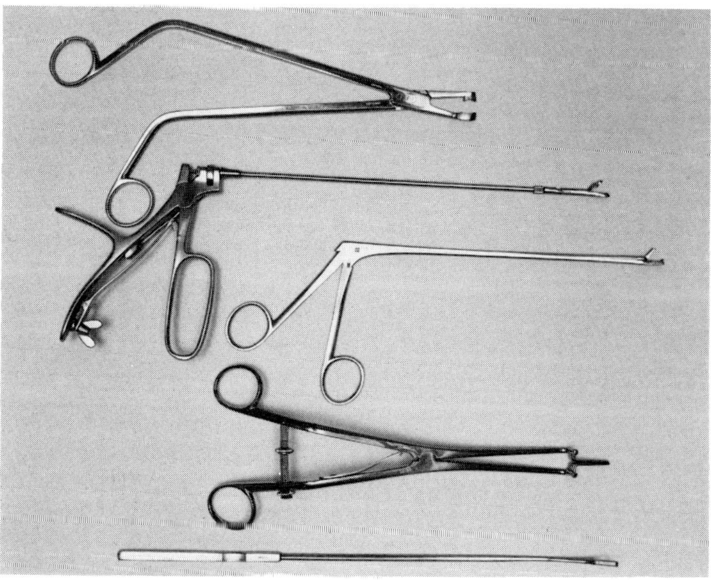

Figure 9. Biopsy instruments (top to bottom): Tischler biopsy forceps, Eppendorfer biopsy forceps, Younge- Kevorkian biopsy forceps, Kogan-Martin endocervical speculum, Kevorkian endocervical curette.

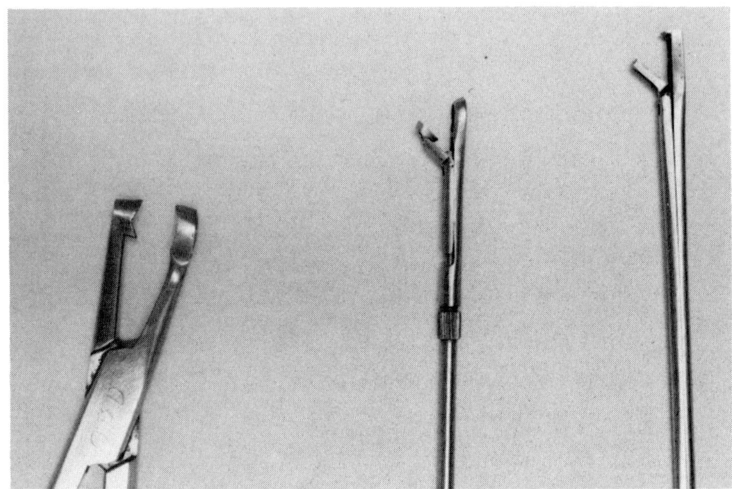

Figure 10. Biopsy instruments, close-up view of heads (l to r): Tischler, Eppendorfer, and Younge-Kevorkian biopsy forceps.

quires a longer waiting time to allow for the appearance of epithelial lesions. The stronger solutions delineate lesions more rapidly but are quite irritating to mucous membranes, especially after repeated applications.

Observable changes in epithelial surfaces are transient ones. They develop within one minute after application of 3 percent acetic acid and fade in two to three minutes. They can be restored with additional acetic acid, and several applications may be required during the course of a single examination.

Inspection of the unprepared cervix and vagina should be followed immediately by scrutiny of the same areas treated with acetic acid. Gauze swabs or cotton-wool pledgets saturated with acetic acid can be used to paint the entire surface of the cervix and adjacent vagina. A liberal application of acetic acid is required. Fine cotton tipped applicators moistened with acetic acid should be used to paint the epithelium of the endocervical canal. The Kogan-Martin endocervical speculum, with a self-retaining attachment located between the handles, permits gentle exposure of the endocervical canal (Figs. 9 and 10). This speculum is especially recommended for use when cervical lesions extend into the endocervical canal. With the aid of an endocervical speculum, at least 1.5 cm of the endocervical canal can be observed in most patients; in many parous individuals, the entire endocervical canal can be seen (Fig. 11).

Tissue treated with acetic acid should be inspected under 5× to 16× magnification. If abnormal vessels are seen, better contrast is achieved by using the green filter and by increasing magnification to 25× or even 40×.

Unlike saline washing, acetic acid washing permits evaluation of changes in tissue color, opacity, and surface contour. Some investigators have suggested that vascular architecture is best observed with saline washing. However, acetic acid application also delineates vascular patterns well. Repeated application of acetic acid sometimes results in substantial dilatation of blood vessels. Abnormal blood vessels which appear following several applications of acetic acid may be iatrogenic.

Iodine Staining

Many colposcopists initially advised that iodine staining of vaginal and cervical mucosa marks the end-point of every colposcopic examination. Solutions traditionally available for this purpose include Schiller (1 gm pure iodine and 2 gm KI in 300 ml H_2O) and Lugol (5 percent iodine and 10 percent KI in H_2O) stains. Ordinarily, native squamous epithelium, high in glycogen content, stains deep mahogany brown when iodine is applied to it. Such an area is referred as Schiller negative or iodine positive. Columnar epithelium, undifferentiated metaplastic epithelium, and abnormal epithelium, in general, are nonglycogenated and therefore do not stain with iodine.

Many colposcopists now agree that the iodine test adds little or nothing to the evaluation of the colposcopic picture. It destroys all minute details necessary for precise diagnosis. It inter-

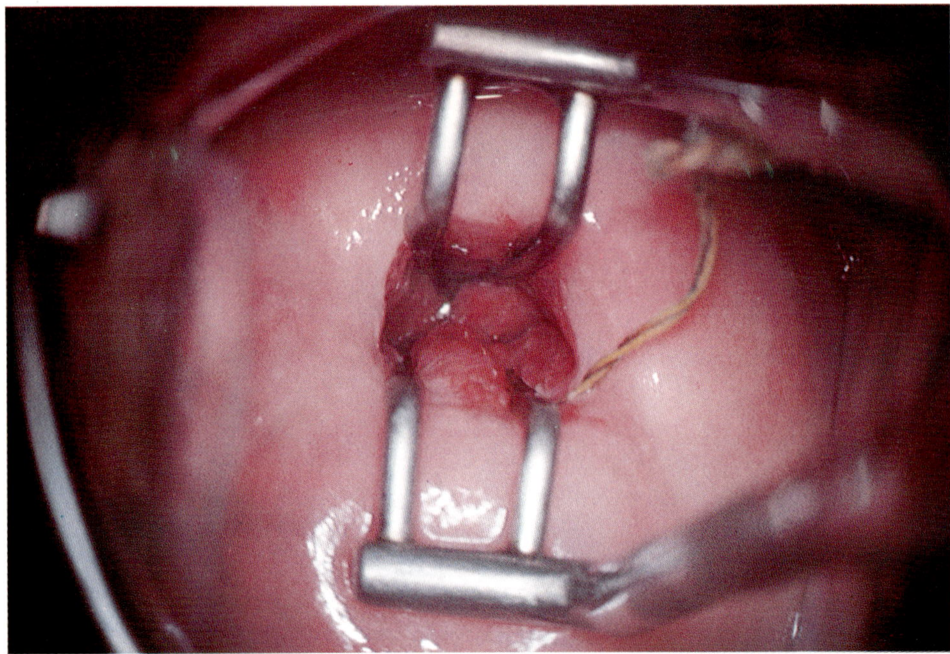

Figure 11. Colpophotograph demonstrating the use of the Kogan-Martin endocervical speculum (8×). The endocervical canal can be seen for a distance of approximately 1.5 cm. Note that the original columnar epithelium within the endocervical canal is flatter than original columnar epithelium on the cervical portio.

feres with localization of the most abnormal areas within a lesion requiring biopsy. Moreover, iodine staining constitutes a nonspecific test. Some malignant tissue may contain glycogen and take up stain. Alternatively, many benign areas—metaplastic epithelium, columnar epithelium, inflammatory changes, vaginal adenosis—all may produce iodine negative areas.

Iodine solutions, if they are used, must be aqueous. An alcohol base causes destruction of tissue which hinders the histologic evaluation of biopsies. Lugol solution is more reliable for colposcopic examination than Schiller solution; the effect of the latter is counteracted by the presence of acetic acid. It is important to keep in mind, however, that all staining techniques fail to distinguish the relative, subtle degrees of atypicality which are essential to the concept of the directed biopsy.

BIOPSY

Colposcopy establishes the location and extent of foci of abnormal epithelium. Colposcopic features such as color, opacity, vascular pattern, and surface contour are reliable indicators of the degree of histologic atypia. Tissue sampling of specific abnormal areas can be performed easily under colposcopic guidance. A biopsy taken in the area of greatest colposcopic abnormality will yield the diagnostic information necessary for implementation of appropriate therapy.

Frequent biopsy during the early part of training in colposcopy is a prerequisite to achieving a clear understanding of the underlying tissue structure. Multiple biopsies, even of seemingly normal areas, properly labeled, provide the best form of instruction by which each colposcopist learns to correlate specific colposcopic pictures with benign, precancerous, or malignant histologic patterns.

Instruments

Carefully excised, well preserved, and oriented, rapidly fixed specimens afford the best opportunity for accurate diagnosis. A variety of instruments may be used for punching out small sections of epithelium. The common biopsy instruments include the Eppendorfer, Kevorkian, Tischler, and Younge forceps. The Eppendorfer forceps takes small, relatively superficial biopsies, whereas the Tischler forceps is designed to extract somewhat larger and deeper tissue sections. The Kevorkian and Younge forceps have serrations on the posterior blade which aid in stabilizing an area requiring biopsy. Care should be taken so that the cutting edges of the biopsy forceps are not dulled by misuse. Forceps should not be autoclaved; they should be soaked in Cidex or sterilized with gas.

Sometimes the tissue of the cervix or vagina is so firm or taut that it cannot be grasped with biopsy forceps. A tonsil or iris hook can be used to tent the epithelium in order to facilitate extraction of a punch biopsy. The iris hook also helps move the cervix away to examine the vaginal fornices. Patients with positive cytologic smears require careful inspection of the vaginal fornices before any definitive treatment is carried out.

It is advisable to obtain biopsy instruments of 15 cm length when colposcopes with fixed working distance of approximately 20 cm are used. Ideally, biopsies should be obtained under colposcopic observation. If the length of a biopsy instrument is greater than 15 cm, the colposcope may need to be removed at the time of biopsy and repositioned to check that a biopsy was removed from the specific area in question.

Technique

The punch biopsy is used primarily for purposes of diagnosis. When taken from the vagina or cervix, such biopsies require no anaesthesia. Punch biopsies may serve as a form of treatment when lesions are small and all borders well defined. Such lesions can be irradicated locally by one or more small bites.

Biopsies should be taken to a depth sufficient to obtain enough stroma for differential diagnosis. The epithelium must be cut at right angles to the surface in order to avoid producing tangential sections. All biopsy forceps should possess openings in the jaws to receive the specimens rather than to compress them; any crushing of the epithelium will cause distortion of the tissue architecture.

Biopsies can be submitted to pathology floating free in separately labeled jars of formalin. In order to conserve jars and space, several specimens can be placed within the same container if each specimen is individually wrapped and labeled. A specimen can be folded in a piece of filter paper or sandwiched between two pieces of thin styrofoam which are held together with paper clips or staples (Fig. 8). Specimens must never be placed in saline; saline destroys surface epithelium and precludes histologic diagnosis.

Several punch biopsies may be required from a single patient. Biopsies at the periphery of the cervix and on the posterior lip should be obtained prior to those at the external os or on the anterior lip. Biopsies from the posterior vaginal wall should be taken before those from the lateral or anterior vaginal surfaces. This system prevents blood from earlier biopsy sites from hampering vision needed for succeeding biopsies.

If bleeding occurs, hemostasis can be achieved by applying Monsel's solution (ferric subsulfate) followed by the gentle pressure of a vaginal tampon. In rare instances, sutures or Weck or Codman clips may be required. Except in cases where the entire area of colposcopic atypicality has been excised and the diagnosis well established, the use of hot cautery at the base of the biopsy site to alleviate bleeding is clearly contraindicated. Cautery destroys surrounding tissue and renders it unsuitable for later histologic or colposcopic examination.

Excisional biopsy and endocervical curettage can be performed under colposcopic observation. The former requires a scalpel and some form of local anesthesia. Excisional biopsy is especially suited to diagnosis of vulvar lesions. It is also useful for treatment of abnormal colposcopic areas on the vagina and cervix when these areas are well demarcated and entirely visible. Endocervical curettage is performed with a Novak or Kevorkian curette (Fig. 9). It has been proposed for use particularly when lesions extend into the endocervical canal. In general, cervical conization or endocervical biopsy provides more reliable diagnostic information than endocervical curettage. Curettings rarely yield tissue with stroma attached; such architectural integrity is needed for histologic diagnosis. Endocervical biopsy can be accomplished with the bronchial biting forceps whose cutting edge is at right angles to the instrument handle. A portion of endocervical tissue with stroma can sometimes be included in a cervical biopsy if the large Tischler forceps are used.

RECORDING DATA

Precise recording of data is an essential element of good colposcopic technique. Sequential photographic studies are desirable; they permit the most accurate analysis of tissue changes related to time.

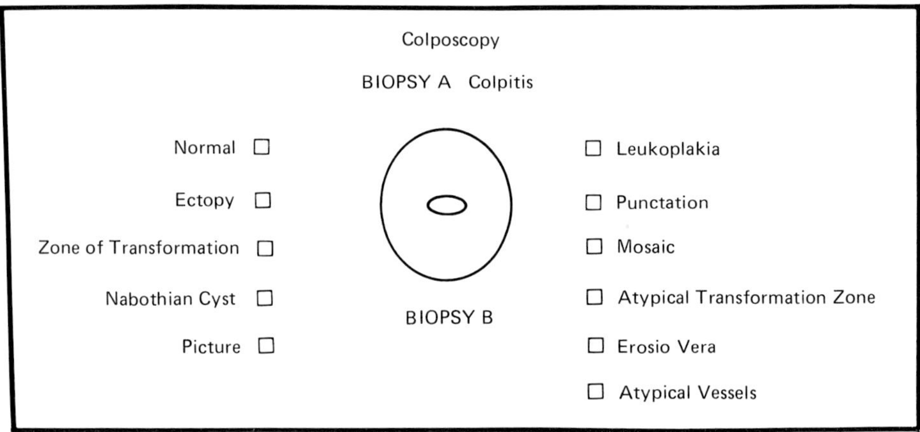

Figure 12. Odell diagram. The size and location of the colposcopic findings can be simply drawn on the diagram and the specific colposcopic lesion can be designated by checking the appropriate square. (Reproduced from Acta Cytol. 13:305, 1968, with permission from Lester D. Odell, M.D.)

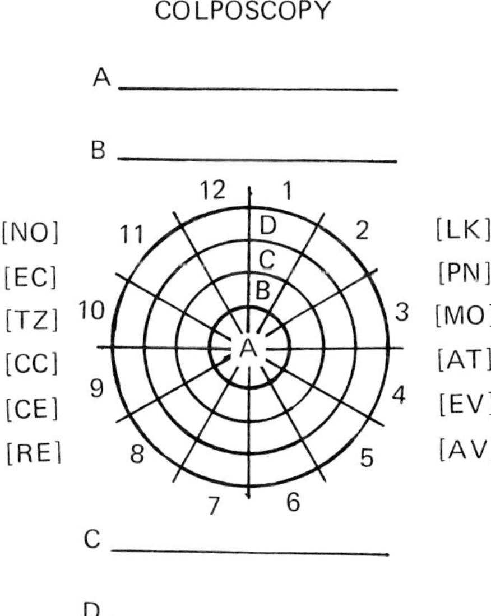

Figure 13. Hammond graph of cervix. NO = Normal; EC = Ectopy; ZT = Transformation zone; CC = Cystic cervicitis; CE = Cervicitis (infectious); RE = Regeneration of tissue; LK = Keratosis, PN = Punctation; MO =Mosaic; AT = Atypical transformation zone; EV = Erosia vera; AV = Atypical vessel

A systematic method such as the Odell diagram for succinct, verbal recording of data is mandatory (Fig. 12). The Hammond graph affords another simple way of keeping records of colposcopic findings and biopsy sites (Fig. 13). It is composed of a series of concentric circles divided into multiple sections. The diagram is available on a rubber stamp and is readily affixed to the medical record.

When video tapes or photographic slides are used to demonstrate precise colposcopic appearances, simple hand drawings along with a clear explanation and list of biopsy sites is probably sufficient for the office or clinic medical record.

3

INDICATIONS

Colposcopy is an adjunctive diagnostic tool. It serves as a companion to the acknowledged laboratory aids of cytology and histopathology for purposes of tissue analysis. Colposcopy is used for selecting the sites of abnormal epithelium for biopsy in patients with abnormal Papanicolaou smears. It is helpful in defining tumor extension and for evaluating benign lesions. It has proved to be valuable for examining and following diethylstilbestrol-exposed offspring. Moreover, it provides an objective basis for teaching as well as for clinical and investigative research (Table 2).

LOCALIZATION OF LESIONS FOR BIOPSY

Colposcopy possibly has its greatest use in evaluating a patient with an abnormal Papanicolaou test. Many patients with positive or doubtful Papanicolaou smears exhibit no obvious target lesion on gross examination with the unaided eye. The challenged benefit of colposcopy is in its potential to help identify and localize with a high degree of accuracy lesions not visible by gross inspection. Directed biopsies of these targeted sites can then be taken. Colposcopic examination ensures that biopsy specimens obtained in this way represent the most advanced histologic process present. Once one has located the areas of

Table 2. Value of colposcopy in gynecology

1. Supplements cytology
2. Determines biopsy sites
3. Evaluates extent of disease
4. Defines vaginal involvement prior to conization or hysterectomy for carcinoma in situ of the cervix
5. Evaluates females exposed to diethylstilbestrol in utero
6. Evaluates lesions of the vagina
7. Evaluates lesions of the vulva
8. Aids in followup of postirradiation change, adenosis, dysplasia, etc.

abnormality and identified the points of greatest cellular atypia by colposcopy, one can remove such loci in whole or in part under continued colposcopic guidance. This can be accomplished usually in an office setting and without anesthesia.

The colposcopically directed biopsy has supplanted some less reliable techniques for localizing atypical lesions. The false negative rate of four quadrant random punch biopsy, for example, is reported to be 12 to 33 percent. The false negative rate of multiple blind biopsies from Schiller nonstaining areas approaches 3 to 8 percent. Cytology, although a practical aid in mass screening for cancer, is obviously of little or no help in pinpointing or delimiting a lesion.

CERVICAL CONIZATION

The advent of colposcopically directed biopsies has obviated the need for at least 80 percent of diagnostic cervical conizations. Although cold knife conization is generally considered a minor surgical procedure, it is not innocuous. Serious complications may result, such as hemorrhage, infection, and infertility. Colposcopy has successfully substituted the safety of the office procedure of directed biopsy for many conizations. Complications of biopsy occur in fewer than 0.1 percent of cases as contrasted with the 10 percent rate of serious hemorrhage and 1 percent additional complications attributable to conization. The major reduction in cervical conization is of special importance for pregnant patients in whom such procedures are associated with much blood loss and frequent fetal wastage. Diagnostic conization in gravidas has been almost entirely eliminated because the squamocolumnar junction in pregnancy is so often everted well out onto the portio of the cervix.

If the entire squamocolumnar junction and part of the endocervical canal are visible with the colposcope, and if the upper limits of any abnormal epithelium are seen, one can feel confident that the areas of maximum colposcopic change will be sampled and subjected to histologic examination; thus, all significant pathology can be diagnosed accurately. When lesions lie wholly within the endocervical canal or extend out of view up into the canal, diagnostic conization is warranted. Since the squamocolumnar junction is visible in its entirety in more than 90 percent of all women, and all or part of the endocervical canal is visible in nearly 75 percent, the need for diagnostic conization is infrequent.

SURGERY AND FOLLOWUP

Colposcopy permits one to delineate the outer limits of tumor on the cervix, vagina, and vulva, so that precise and adequate surgical margins can be achieved. When cervical conization is employed for treatment in a young patient with carcinoma in situ of the cervix, colposcopy can help determine appropriate areas for surgical incisions. Approximately 6 percent of early cervical cancers have a cancerous focus or foci in the vaginal fornices as part of a multicentric growth. Colposcopy enables one to recognize these areas preoperatively.

After hysterectomy for cervical or endometrial carcinoma, or subsequent to radiation therapy, followup colposcopy can be used to investigate for the presence and precise location of early vaginal recurrence so that treatment can be carried out expeditiously.

BENIGN DISEASE

Colposcopy is useful in determining the nature of benign disease. It helps to distinguish preclinical carcinoma from important benign conditions such as condylomata acuminata, papillomata, and trichomonas vaginalis vaginitis, all of which may give rise to abnormal cytology. In the presence of a negative Papanicolaou smear, many benign changes are more readily diagnosed with colposcopy than by speculum examination. Unnecessary biopsies of benign lesions can therefore be avoided.

DIETHYLSTILBESTROL EXPOSURE

Serial colposcopy appears to be the most effective method for evaluating the epithelium of the vagina and cervix in patients exposed in utero to diethylstilbestrol (DES). The benign condition of vaginal adenosis is observed with the colposcope in approximately 90 percent of DES offspring. It is seen with Lugol staining in only 40 to 60 percent of cases; it cannot be definitively identified by gross or cytologic examination.

The potential for development of clear cell adenocarcinoma or squamous cell dysplasia of the vagina in these patients is the primary subject of concern. Foci of adenosis in the upper vagina of DES exposed patients is submucosal in location in 60 percent, and no exfoliation can be expected to occur in these cases. Thus, dysplastic or neoplastic transformation may be undetected by cytology at least 60 percent of the time. Moreover, some cases of clear cell adenocarcinoma have demonstrated negative cytology. Hopefully, microscopic foci of invasive clear cell adenocarcinoma or preclinical squamous carcinoma will be detected with the colposcope long before they are visible to the naked eye. One anticipates that any changes in the morphology of the epithelium which are noted by serial colposcopy may signal the presence of malignant disease.

TEACHING AND RESEARCH

Colposcopy is valuable for teaching and clinical research. It has created for students and clinicians a new dimension to the understanding of the pathogenesis of neoplasia by providing a unique means of observing and evaluating tissue in the process of dynamic change. The colposcope has enabled investigators to establish protocols for treatment of dysplastic and neoplastic lesions by local excision or local destruction by electrodiathermy or cryosurgery. Carbon dioxide laser treatments have been used on an experimental basis as a method for eradicating lesions of the cervix and vagina. Such lasers are constructed for use only when attached to a colposcope.

4

HISTOLOGIC BASIS OF COLPOSCOPY

Every colposcopic picture is the counterpart of a specific tissue pattern (Fig. 14). Each tissue pattern, in turn, is determined by the nature of its surface epithelium and associated connective tissue stroma. The colposcope produces its effect by illuminating both surface epithelium and underlying stroma. When a sheet of epithelium composed of a particular cell population is interposed between the colposcopic light source and subjacent stroma, a characteristic visual impression is created. The visual image observed is a reflection of epithelial cell number, organization, and morphology. This image is also influenced by the vascular arrangement of the underlying stroma. Each of the many variations in stromal vascular architecture can be modified by a number of possible changes in epithelial cellular morphology. The various combinations of epithelium and stroma produce identifiable colposcopic images. Consequently, both normal and abnormal epithelia take on colposcopic appearances almost as characteristic as those seen on histologic examination. Each cervix and vagina is colposcopically unique.

Variations in colposcopic appearances are manifested by changes in morphologic features such as color and opacity, vascular configuration, and surface contour. These features differentiate normal from atypical tissue and form the basis for all colposcopic examination.

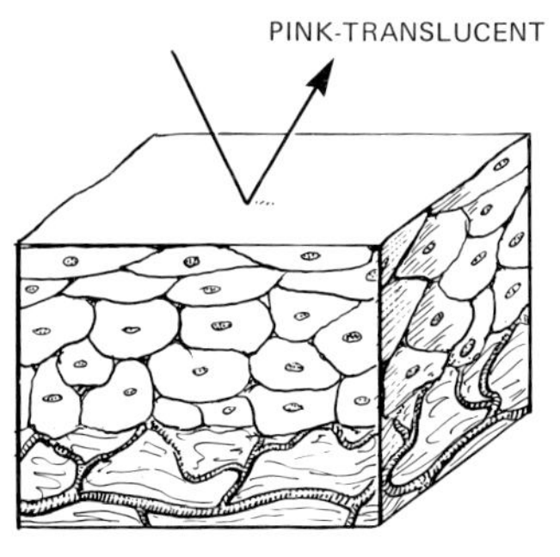

A

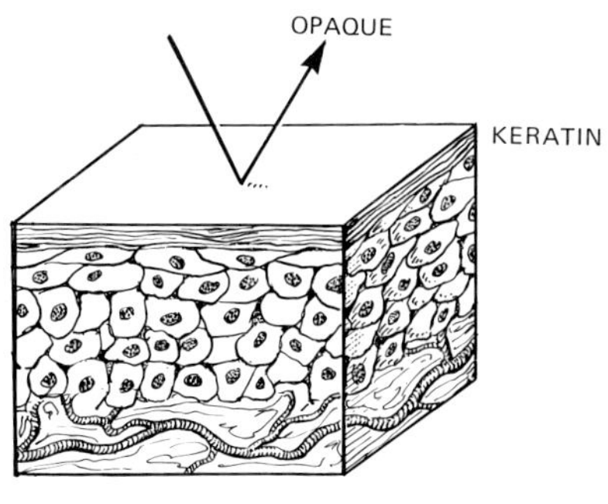

B

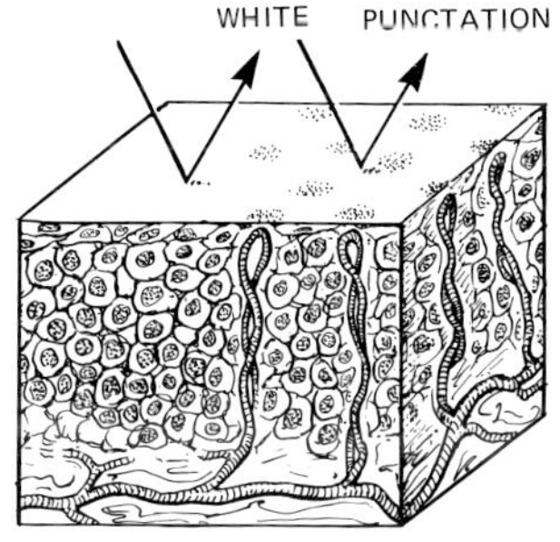

C

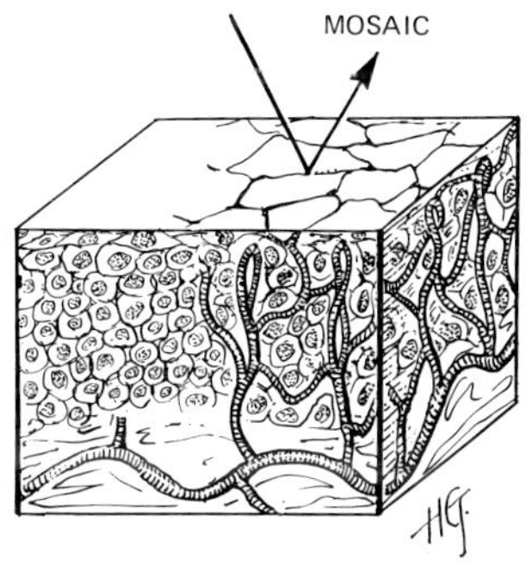

D

Figure 14. Tissue basis of colposcopy. A strip or sheet of epithelium composed of a characteristic cell population intervenes between the light source and the underlying stroma.

COLOR AND OPACITY

Color and opacity are important indicators of the cell population of epithelium. Native squamous epithelium is the term used to refer to the epithelial layer that usually lines the vagina and part of the cervical portio. It appears pink, translucent, and featureless under colposcopic examination. The incident light passes uniformly through several homogeneous squamous cell layers to yield a uniform homogeneous surface pattern.

Native columnar epithelium is the term used to refer to the tissue that lines the endocervical canal. Such tissue is sometimes present also on the exocervix around the anatomic external cervical os. It is composed of only a single layer of cells which overlies a highly vascular stroma. It is usually thrown up into folds. When illuminated by the colposcope, this tissue appears quite red as a result of the transparency of the columnar cells and proximity of the stromal capillary bed to the epithelial surface. The red color is most pronounced when columnar tissue has first been washed with saline. Acetic acid creates the characteristic appearance of grape clusters because of cellular edema which increases the surface opacity and tends to reduce the color contrast.

Specific properties, such as epithelial height, cell density, nuclear atypia, cellular differentiation, and mucus or keratin production, alter the optical response. Any condition which exhibits hyperchromatic nuclei, diminished cytoplasm, or dense keratin accumulation reflects more light than normal tissue and therefore appears opaque or white under the colposcope. Inflammation can alter the color of normal squamous epithelium by increasing vascularity, keratin production, and so forth. Surface tissue comprised of fewer than normal squamous cell layers transmits more light and thus appears more translucent than native squamous epithelium which is typically 15 to 20 cell thicknesses. Postmenopausal squamous epithelium is especially pale because of a decrease in stromal vascularity along with a decrease in epithelial cell density and nuclear size. The thinness and relative colposcopic translucency of epithelium can be offset by the increased nuclear density of undifferentiated cells. A strip of epithelium which displays fewer than normal layers of cells with larger than normal nuclear size may create the same opaque colposcopic appearance as tissue which is composed of many cell layers and small nuclei.

VASCULAR CONFIGURATION

One of the principal advantages of colposcopy is its capability for evaluating surface and subepithelial vascular structure and spatial arrangement. This aspect of tissue analysis is virtually indiscernable by histologic sections. Tissues which differ in cellular structure and activity show important differences in number, size, configuration, calibre, and disposition of their vessels. Variation in the vascular architecture of adjacent tissues permits clear distinction between physiologic and pathologic areas of vaginal and cervical epithelium.

Specific types of terminal vessels are characteristic of the normal vaginal and cervical epithelia. Vessels within the villi of columnar epithelium are not easily delineated with a colposcope; columnar tissue appears uniformly red because of the delicate quality of the stromal vasculature which is located at the same uniform depth in all areas. Capillary patterns in the form of network or hairpin structures are basic to native squamous epithelium. When connective tissue papillae of the squamous epithelium of the cervix and vagina are poorly developed or absent, the stromal vasculature is flattened and everywhere equidistant from the tissue surface. Consequently, a meshwork or network of delicate capillaries is seen. Atrophic squamous epithelium, because it is especially translucent, sometimes displays spider-like vessels beneath the network capillaries.

Hairpin capillaries are observed if stromal papillae are well developed in squamous epithelium. A hairpin vessel is formed by the ascending and descending branches of a capillary loop within a papilla. The extent of stromal papillation and the angle of observation determine whether or not such hairpin structures are seen in their entirety. Within the same colposcopic section, hairpin vessels can be viewed tangentially as crests of loops, or directly on end as fine punctation vessels.

Pathologic epithelia also demonstrate characteristic vascular patterns based on changes in vessel number, size, organization, intercapillary distance, and so forth. Their evolution will be discussed in relation to the development of the atypical transformation zone.

SURFACE CONTOUR

Alterations in surface contour reflect growth disorders of epithelium, specifically potential neoplasia. The stereoscopic magnification provided by the colposcope lends itself to the effective study of surface configurations. Native squamous epithelium has a smooth surface, whereas columnar epithelium has multiple grape-like papillomatous excrescences. The "grapes" or villi are most prominent at the distal end of the endocervical canal and often circumorally on the exposed exocervix. In situ and invasive carcinomas can both display raised and irregular surfaces; dysplasias rarely do.

It should be emphasized that all colposcopic appearances are based on the morphologic criteria described above. Each colposcopic pattern reflects its associated histologic structure.

5

DEVELOPMENT OF THE NORMAL TRANSFORMATION ZONE

The visible portion of the female genital tract is covered by stratified squamous epithelium which lines the vagina and exocervix and simple columnar epithelium which lines the endocervical canal. The junction of these two tissue types (the squamocolumnar junction) can occur at various locations on the uterine cervix. The squamocolumnar junction commonly coincides with the anatomic external cervical os. In postmenopausal females, it occurs frequently within the endocervical canal. Most menstruating females display this junction on the exposed exocervix. When this occurs, it is often mistakenly referred to as a cervical eversion, ectropion, congenital erosion, or erythroplakia. It is present in many female fetuses. It occurs at other times of life in exaggerated form in response to high estrogen stimuli, such as puberty, pregnancy, or oral contraceptives. In approximately 4 percent of the female population and in many women who were exposed to diethylstilbestrol in utero, the squamocolumnar junction may actually extend out onto the vaginal fornices or vaginal wall.

The squamous tissues of the vagina and cervix are designated colposcopically as the original or native squamous epithelium; the columnar tissue is called the original or native columnar epithelium. Native squamous epithelium shows little variation

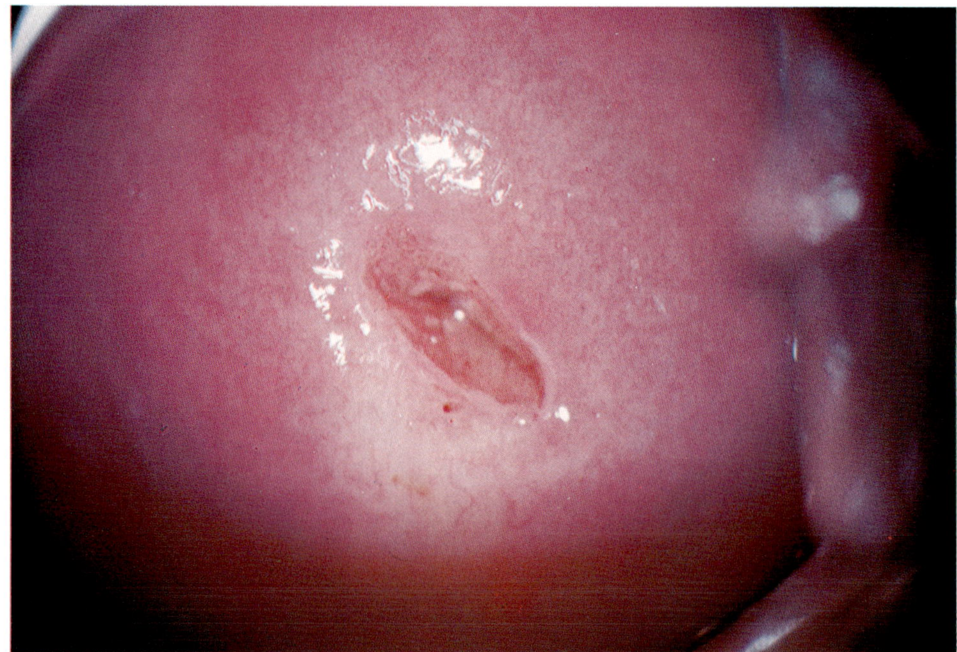

Figure 15. Colpophotograph of a normal cervix demonstrating native stratified squamous epithelium with feathery vascular arrangement (12.5×). Note the columnar epithelium at the external cervical os.

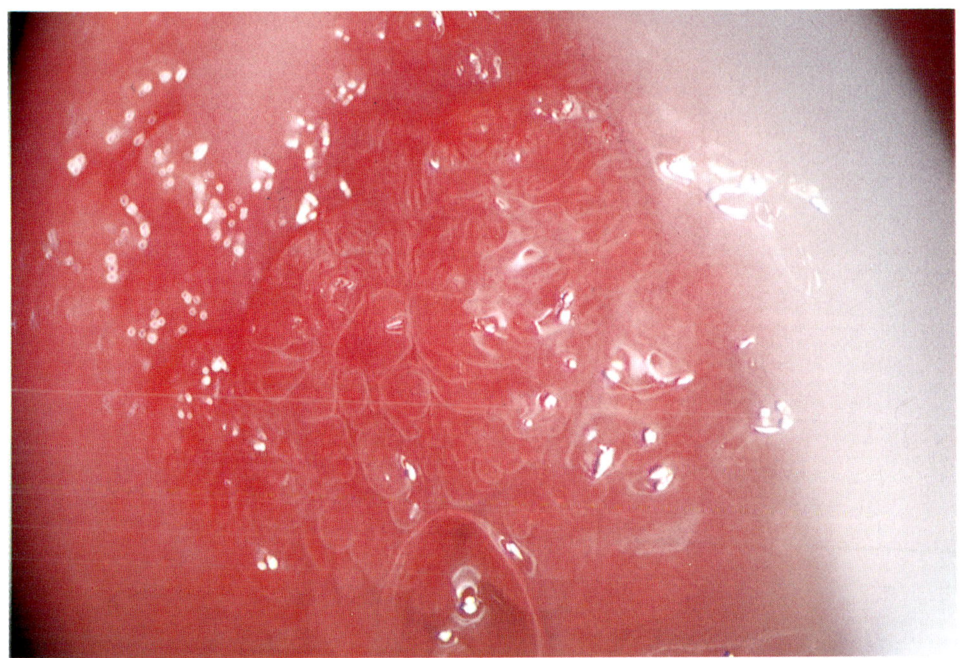

Figure 16. Colpophotograph of a normal cervix demonstrating the grape-like structure of native columnar epithelium (20×).

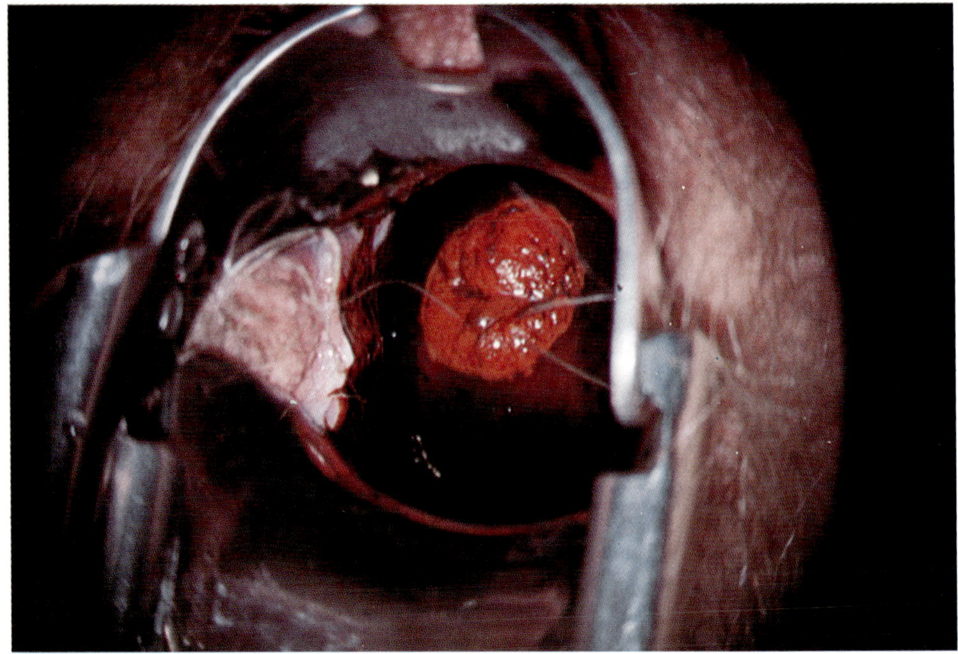

Figure 17. Colpophotograph of a normal cervix stained with Lugol's iodine (8×). Note that original stratified squamous epithelium takes the stain whereas original columnar epithelium does not.

from subject to subject. Under the colposcope, it is uniformly pale pink and translucent and frequently exhibits a feathery vascular arrangement (Fig. 15). Native columnar epithelium is unmistakable colposcopically. It is readily identified by its intense red hue and multiple grape-like projections or villi (Fig. 16). Each villus possesses a single looped capillary which is sometimes seen colposcopically, especially with the use of the green filter. Columnar epithelium, in contrast to squamous epithelium, usually fails to stain with iodine (Fig. 17).

The colposcopic examination is directed primarily toward investigating the tissue in the area where original squamous and original columnar epithelia come together. At this squamocolumnar interface, columnar epithelium is gradually transformed into squamous epithelium by a process of metaplasia. This dynamic area of change is known as the "transformation zone" (Fig. 18). The transformation zone is the principal focus of colposcopic interest. A clear concept of the transformation zone is essential for understanding the origin and development of cervical neoplasia. It is within this location specifically that preclinical squamous cancer and epithelial dysplasias are believed to develop.

The junction between original columnar and original squamous epithelium is transitory. Presumably as a result of high plasma estrogen concentration and low pH conditions of the vagina, the original columnar epithelium becomes replaced by metaplastic squamous epithelium. The original squamocolumnar junction is therefore converted into a squamo-squamo junction of original and metaplastic squamous tissue. A new squamocolumnar junction occurs between the original columnar epithelium and the transformed areas. This junction may then be subject to a similar transformation process at a later time.

The process of metaplasia is multifocal. Metaplastic squamous epithelium is often identified at the outer edge of columnar epithelium adjacent to squamous tissue. It also frequently develops as discrete islands within the columnar tissue (Fig. 19).

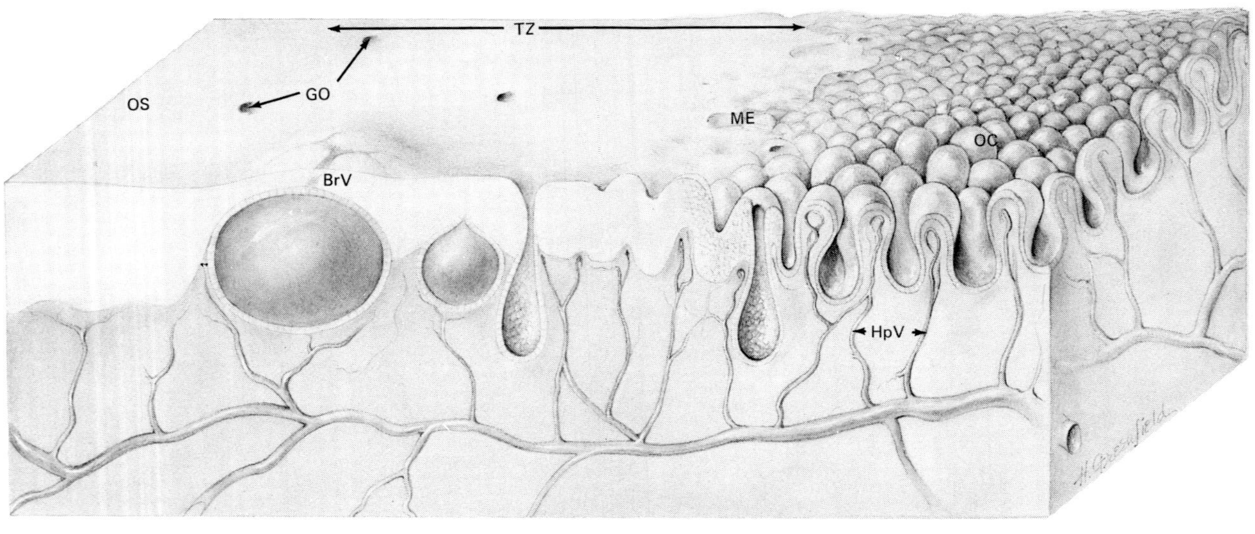

Figure 18. Development of the normal transformation zone. Diagram representing the process of metaplasia from columnar to stratified squamous epithelium producing the transformation zone. (Modified from René Cartier.) OC = Original columnar epithelium; HpV = Hairpin blood vessel within papillae of columnar epithelium; ME = Area of early metaplasia; TZ = Transformation zone; BrV = Blood vessels over nabothian cyst; GO = Gland openings; OS = Original stratified squamous epithelium

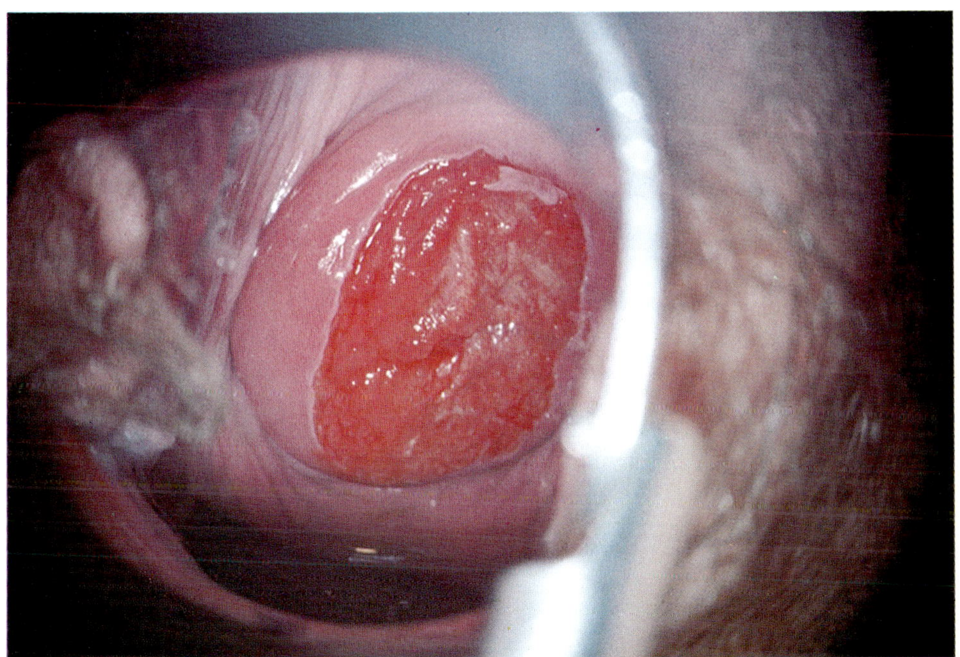

Figure 19. Colpophotograph of the portio of the cervix showing an island of metaplasia within the columnar epithelium at 1 o'clock position (12.5×).

The many metaplastic foci gradually widen, coalesce, and eventually join the peripheral component. Since abnormal epithelium can arise from metaplastic tissue, multifocal areas of metaplasia can obviously give rise to multifocal atypical change.

The normal physiologic transition from columnar to squamous epithelium occurs throughout the female lifetime. It is most active at three phases of life: (1) fetal existence and neonatal period, (2) menarche, and (3) first pregnancy. The periods of most active metaplasia appear to correspond to the times at which high levels of estrogen are present. Estrogen stimulation enhances cervical eversion and allows a maximal amount of columnar tissue to be exposed to the vaginal environment. Estrogen promotes an acid pH in the vagina; this acidity appears to initiate the metaplastic process.

During fetal existence, menarche, and first pregnancy, metaplasia is active in its early and immature form. Metaplasia at other times is minimal. Active metaplasia in the fetus takes place late in pregnancy (primarily from 28 weeks to term) and has been attributed to the influence of maternal steroids. After birth, metaplasia slackens, probably as a result of the diminished level of plasma steroids and neutral vaginal secretion in the neonate. With the surge of estrogen that occurs at the menarche and during the first pregnancy, the transformation process is reactivated. Patients taking oral contraceptives, although often displaying large cervical eversions, demonstrate a remarkably slow process of metaplasia. This is probably due to the protection afforded by the increased amount of cervical mucus. Metaplasia can be promoted by the use of contraceptive jellies because of their markedly acid pH.

Complete transformation from columnar to squamous epithelium occurs over a period of many years. The process of metaplasia may be divided into three stages:

1. Early metaplasia
2. Well developed metaplasia

3. Fully developed metaplasia (gland openings, nabothian follicles, typical vascular patterns)

The process of metaplasia results in the development of a new squamous epithelium which is at first immature. When it reaches maturity it does not seem subject to cancer formation. Mature metaplasia is a permanent change. By contrast, the initial process of metaplasia is vulnerable to genetic change. New squamous cell populations with acquired neoplastic potential can arise from active immature metaplasia. Epithelia which exhibit morphologic characteristics of precursors of squamous cancer are the principal subjects of interest to the colposcopist.

EARLY METAPLASIA

The earliest colposcopic changes of metaplasia involve loss of translucency of the tips of the villi of columnar epithelium along with increase in clarity and demarcation of vascular structures (Fig. 20). Colposcopically, the tips of villi stand out as individual opaque structures against a background of red color. The red color is created by the columnar tissue which remains within the clefts between villi.

Histologically, the tall columnar cells at the tips of the villi are replaced by several layers of low cuboidal cells. The metaplastic squamous epithelium originates from multipotential stromal cells that are found subjacent to the columnar epithelium. These so-called "activated stromal cells" or "columnar reserve cells" become visible (or at least recognizable) only at the moment that the metaplastic process becomes manifest. These cells then become apparent and increase in number before they differentiate. They develop a less densely staining nucleus and increased cytoplasm, are drawn into long processes, and transform into squamous cells.

All metaplasia takes place within the transformation zone. The transformation zone can be quite extensive or very limited; its colposcopic picture is extremely variable according to the ex

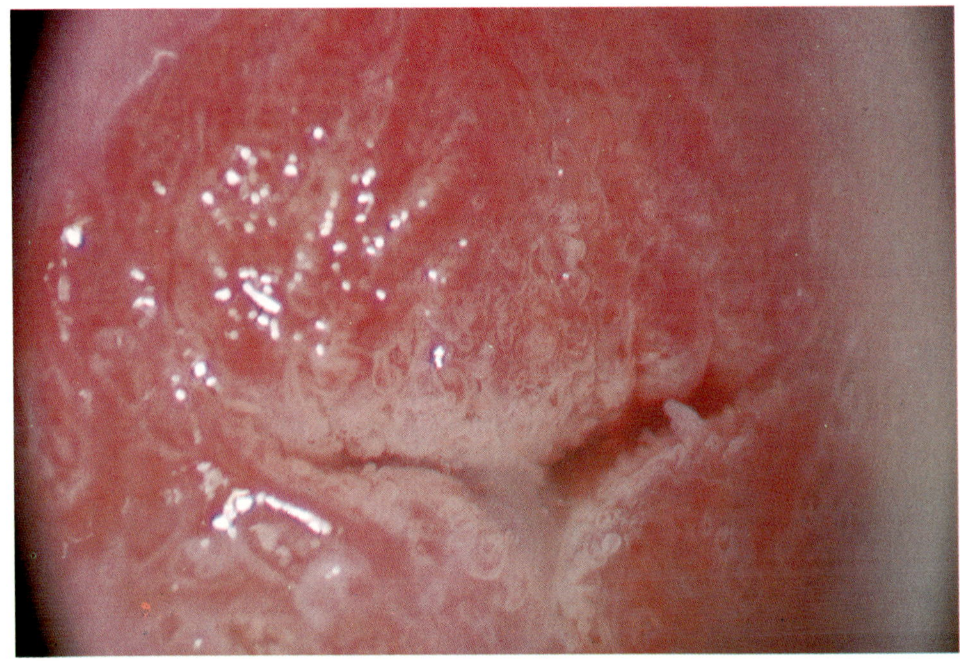

Figure 20. Colpophotograph of columnar epithelium on the exocervix undergoing early metaplasia (20×). Note that adjacent villi are fused with increased opacity of the surface especially at the 11 to 1 o'clock position.

tent of the squamous metaplasia. Sometimes, only a few tongues of squamous metaplasia or isolated areas of squamous metaplasia are visible in the columnar epithelium. Alternatively, the original columnar epithelium can be almost completely covered by metaplastic squamous tissue.

Immature metaplastic squamous epithelium consists of 6 to 8 cell thicknesses of undifferentiated surface cells which undergo a gradual process of maturation. After acetic acid is applied to immature metaplastic squamous epithelium, it becomes more opaque than original squamous epithelium, possibly as a result of the increased nuclear-to-cytoplasmic ratio exhibited by immature squamous cells. Undifferentiated metaplastic epithelium can be difficult to distinguish from dysplasia or carcinoma in situ histologically. Immature metaplastic tissue is nonglycogenated and characteristically iodine negative. As a result, staining techniques are not adequate to distinguish early metaplastic from dysplastic tissue. It must be emphasized that the characteristics of the transformation zone are best recognized by its colposcopic appearance.

WELL DEVELOPED METAPLASIA

As the metaplastic process advances, a multilayered undifferentiated sheet of epithelial cells is gradually formed. The activated stromal cells which cap the villi rapidly divide and extend into the clefts between adjacent villi. The tips of the villi coalesce, and fusion of the opposed surfaces of villi occurs (Fig. 21).

Colposcopically, although individual opaque villi appear fused, minute humps are present on the tissue surface which represent the tips of the old villi. This tissue also is not stained by iodine.

FULLY DEVELOPED METAPLASIA

The end stage of the metaplastic process represents the near obliteration of the original villous structures. A smooth surface of

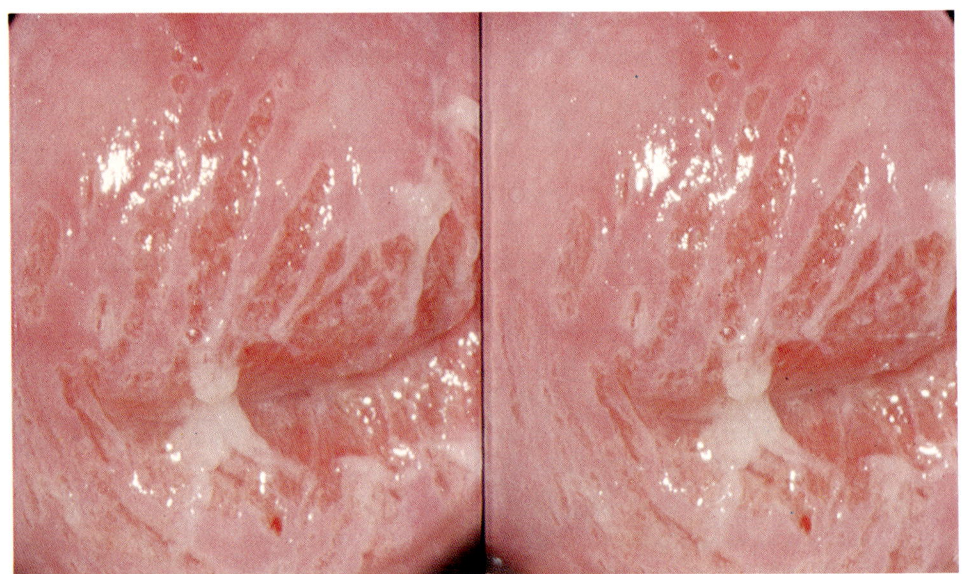

Figure 21. Leisegang stereophotograph of the cervix demonstrating tongues of well developed metaplastic tissue extending into the columnar epithelium toward the external cervical os (13.5×).

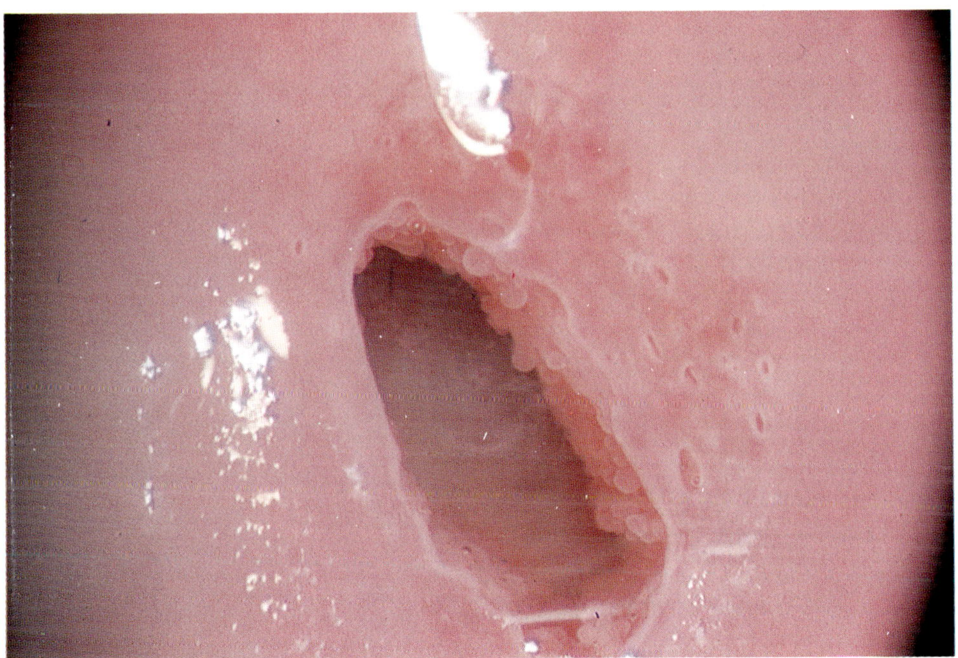

Figure 22. Colpophotograph of fully developed typical transformation zone (20×). Note gland openings on the exocervix. These gland openings are surrounded by smooth stratified squamous epithelium which appears colposcopically like that of original stratified squamous tissue.

multilayered, increasingly differentiated epithelium is produced. The vascular supply remains similar to that of the original squamous epithelium; mature metaplastic tissue exhibits both network and hairpin capillaries of varying number and pattern (Fig. 22). A third type of terminal vessel, not identified in normal squamous tissue, is often seen in typical (i.e., normal) mature transformation zones. This vessel runs parallel with the tissue surface and is strikingly large; it divides dichotomously into a network of delicate capillaries of normal or even increased intercapillary distance. Such vessels are associated with nabothian cysts.

Even in mature transformation zones, the coalescence of villi or papillae is rarely complete. Islands of columnar tissue often remain in the deep clefts within the stroma below the metaplastic epithelium. Such areas can have an outlet to the surface which is surrounded by a narrow band of heaped up squamous epithelium (Fig. 23). Mucus is secreted and expelled through these small gland openings. Under the colposcope, these gland openings appear characteristically as dark red craters encircled by a dense white border. If areas of columnar tissue have no communication with the tissue surface, retention cysts (nabothian cysts) develop. Under the colposcope, these cysts are yellowish and translucent and are elevated above the level of surrounding epithelium (Fig. 24). Large branching blood vessels traverse their surface (Fig. 25).

The ultimate maturity of the metaplastic epithelium is its development into a fully differentiated squamous tissue distinguishable only with difficulty from the native squamous variety. Histologically, it is almost impossible to differentiate between original squamous and mature metaplastic squamous epithelium. Both stain with iodine. Colposcopically, columnar remnants (nabothian follicles and gland openings) serve to define the distal margin of the transformation zone, the original border between native squamous and metaplastic squamous epithelium.

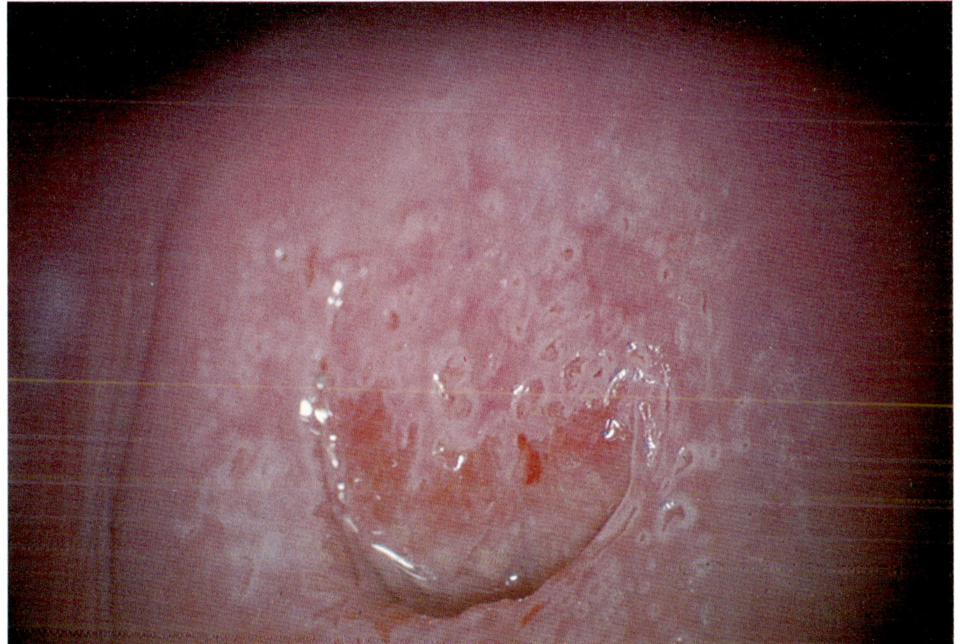

Figure 23. Colpophotograph showing a wide, fully developed transformation zone (12.5×). Note the numerous gland openings each surrounded by a white collar of heaped-up epithelium.

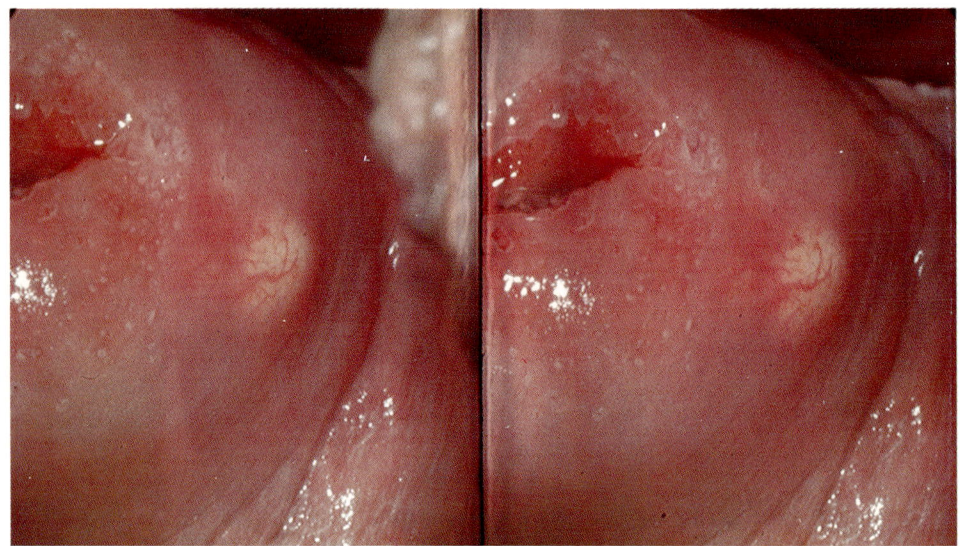

Figure 24. Leisegang stereophotograph of the cervix showing a fully developed transformation zone with a nabothian cyst to the left of the external cervical os (13.5×). Note that the nabothian cyst represents the outer limit of the transformation zone, the initial junction of original columnar and stratified squamous epithelium.

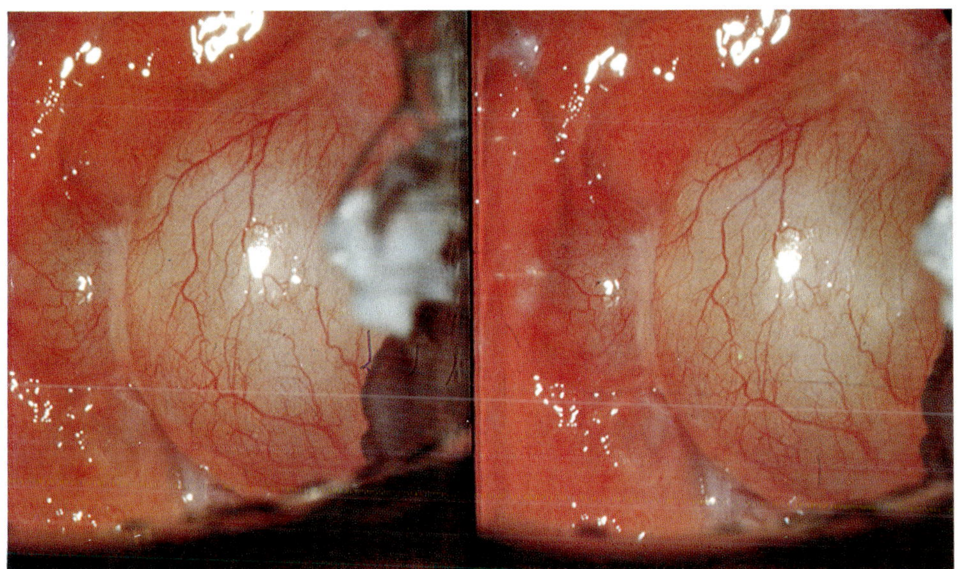

Figure 25. Leisegang colpophotograph showing large nabothian cyst with numerous dichotomizing blood vessels at the surface (13.5×).

The evolution of metaplasia can arrest at any stage to persist as immature tissue throughout life or to await further stimuli to maturation. The mature state, though generally achieved gradually, may be reached early; it has even been observed in some fetuses. At the other extreme, immature forms have been observed in postmenopausal women. The tendency toward maturity is very variable. It imparts to each subject a fingerprint-like individuality.

Table 3. Colposcopic terminology*

Normal Colposcopic Findings
1. Original squamous epithelium
2. Columnar epithelium
3. Transformation zone

Abnormal Colposcopic Findings
1. Atypical transformation zone
   a. White epithelium
   b. Punctation
   c. Nosaic
   d. Keratosis (leukoplakia)
   e. Abnormal blood vessels
2. Suspect frank invasive cancer

Unsatisfactory Colposcopic Findings

Other Colposcopic Findings
1. Vaginocervicitis
2. True erosion
3. Atrophic epithelium
4. Condyloma, papilloma

*The nomenclature for colposcopy was approved by the Committee on Terminology of the Second World Congress of Cervical Pathology and Colposcopy, October 1975, Graz, Austria.

6

THE ATYPICAL TRANSFORMATION ZONE

As a result of the influence of unknown mutagenic agents, areas of metaplastic epithelium within the transformation zone can acquire neoplastic potential. In these areas, columnar epithelium undergoes a process of atypical metaplasia and an atypical transformation zone is created (Fig. 26).

An atypical transformation zone is readily identified colposcopically. Abnormal metaplastic epithelium is characterized by the appearance within the transformation zone of keratosis (previously termed leukoplakia), white epithelium, punctation, mosaic structure, and abnormal blood vessels. These atypical colposcopic tissue patterns may occur singly or in combination; they may be unifocal or multifocal and almost invariably are sharply delineated from surrounding normal tissue. Their lateral margins rarely, if ever, extend beyond the original squamocolumnar junction onto the native squamous epithelium.

With the exception of keratosis, none of the lesions peculiar to the atypical transformation zone can be seen with the naked eye prior to the application of acetic acid. Areas of punctation, mosaic structure, and abnormal blood vessels can sometimes be observed without acetic acid, but not without the magnification provided by the colposcope.

It should be emphasized that the colposcopic variations of

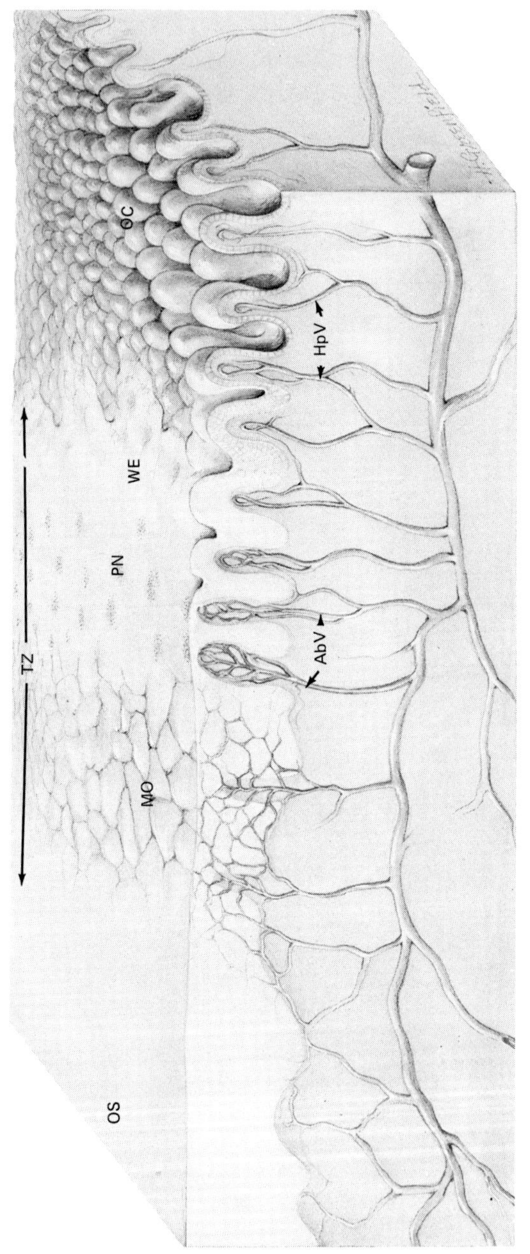

Figure 26. Development of the atypical transformation zone. Diagram representing the process of abnormal metaplasia producing an atypical transformation zone. (Modified from René Cartier.) OC = Original columnar epithelium; HpV = Hairpin blood vessel within papillae of columnar epithelium; TZ = Transformation zone; AbV = Abnormal blood vessel; WE = White epithelium; PN = Punctation; MO = Mosaic; OS = Original stratified squamous epithelium

atypia are found primarily within the transformation zone but can be present also in the vagina and on the vulva. Moreover, the same colposcopic findings that often signal a neoplastic change may occur in non-neoplastic conditions such as normal metaplasia, infection, inflammation, and regeneration and repair following trauma, cautery, or cryosurgery. The presence of an abnormal transformation zone, though highly suggestive, does not prove that neoplasia exists.

WHITE EPITHELIUM

The white focal lesion constitutes the most common appearance of the atypical transformation zone. White epithelium exhibits a flat smooth surface which is level with the surrounding normal tissue. It displays either no visible terminal vessels or only minimally developed vascular structures. Without acetic acid, the white lesion is not evident colposcopically and cannot be distinguished from adjacent normal epithelium (Figs. 27 and 28).

Whiteness of the abnormal epithelium presumably is related to the nuclear predominance of atypical cells. Light is reflected from atypical cells that have dense, hyperchromatic nuclei and scanty cytoplasm, but it is readily transmitted through surrounding normal cells with abundant cytoplasm and homogeneous nuclei. The significance of a white lesion is related to the intensity of its whiteness as well as the sharpness of its borders. The whiter and more distinct the lesion, the greater is its histologic significance. Dysplasia or even in situ carcinoma with high nuclear density and low transparency can produce this appearance.

PUNCTATION AND MOSAIC STRUCTURE

As columnar epithelium undergoes atypical metaplasia, the vascular patterns of punctation and mosaic structure develop. During atypical metaplasia, papillae do not coalesce or fuse with each other as they do during the normal metaplastic process. Ultimately, a flat sheet of stroma covered by uniformly

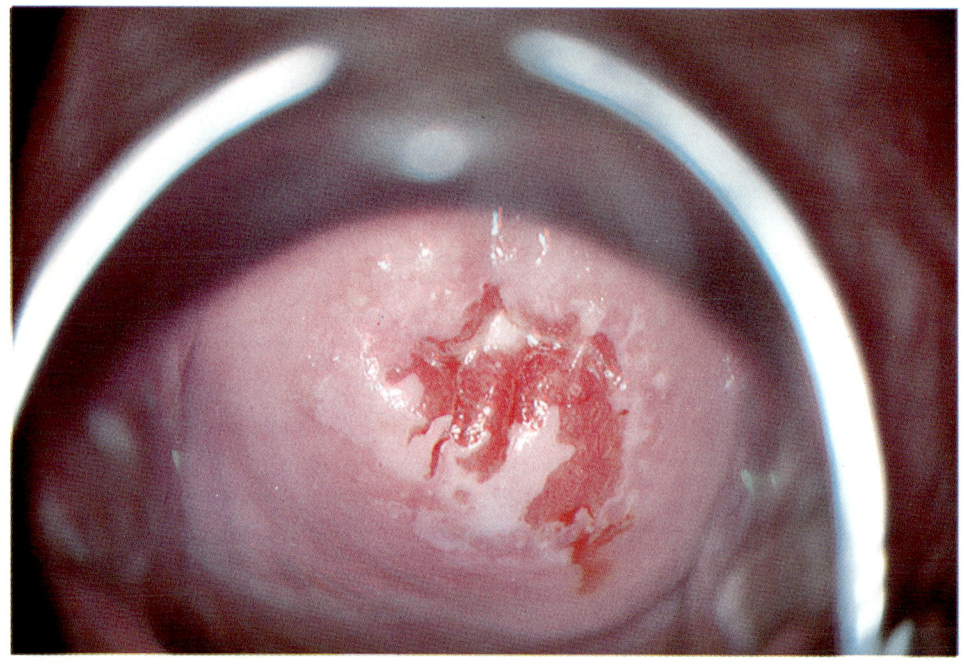

Figure 27. Colpophotograph of the cervix of a 27-year-old nulligravida referred for evaluation of abnormal Papanicolaou smears of 1.5 years duration. Photo taken prior to application of acetic acid (8×). Note that no lesion is visible on the portio of the cervix.

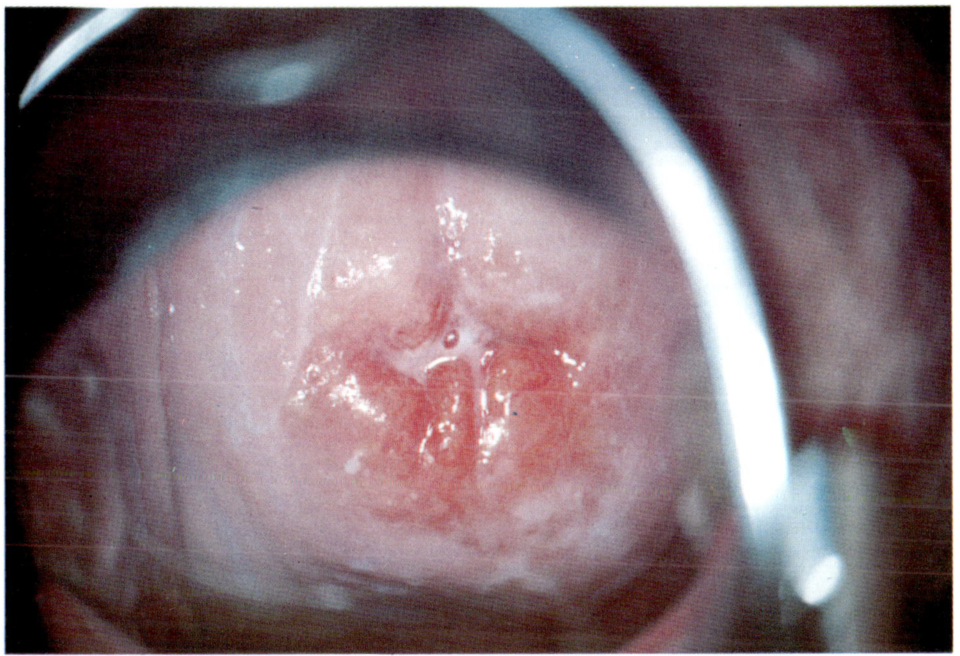

Figure 28. Colpophotograph of the cervix seen in Fig. 27 following application of acetic acid (8×). Note the well circumscribed white focal lesion present on the posterior lip of the cervix. Biopsy of this area revealed severe dysplasia.

distributed metaplastic squamous epithelium is not produced. Instead, the vascular network within each villus persists and undergoes marked proliferation. The central vascular network of these remaining stromal papillae features blood vessel loops which extend close to the surface of the overlying epithelium. Consequently, the blood supply of the surface epithelium is greater in atypical than in normal transformation zones. Punctation and mosaic patterns are reflections of this abnormal developmental process (Fig. 29).

Colposcopically in very early forms of atypical metaplasia, after the application of acetic acid, the stromal papillae appear as reddish fields surrounded by white strands of metaplastic epithelium. This appearance has been called "reverse mosaic." The red islands represent the tops of the stromal papillae (with underlying superficial vascularity) and the white strands are produced by a piling up of atypical metaplastic squamous cells which invade and fill surrounding clefts and folds. Since connective tissue papillae become thinner and cleft areas widen as the atypical metaplastic process advances, this colposcopic picture is very short lived (its duration is approximately 14 days) and therefore is seldom observed.

Progression of atypical metaplasia is characterized by increased proliferative activity of the squamous epithelium within the clefts and lateral compression of the stromal papillae. The hairpin or looped vessels within the papillae may undergo dilatation and proliferation near the surface or may form ramifications around buds of atypical epithelium. In the first instance, capillaries form a stippled pattern and the lesion appears colposcopically as punctation; in the second case, a mosaic structure is observed. Since the processes of development of mosaic and punctation patterns from original columnar epithelium are basically very similar, both tissue types frequently are found in the same focal lesion (Fig. 30).

Colposcopically, punctation and mosaic terminal vessels may show wide variations in size, shape, mutual arrangement, and

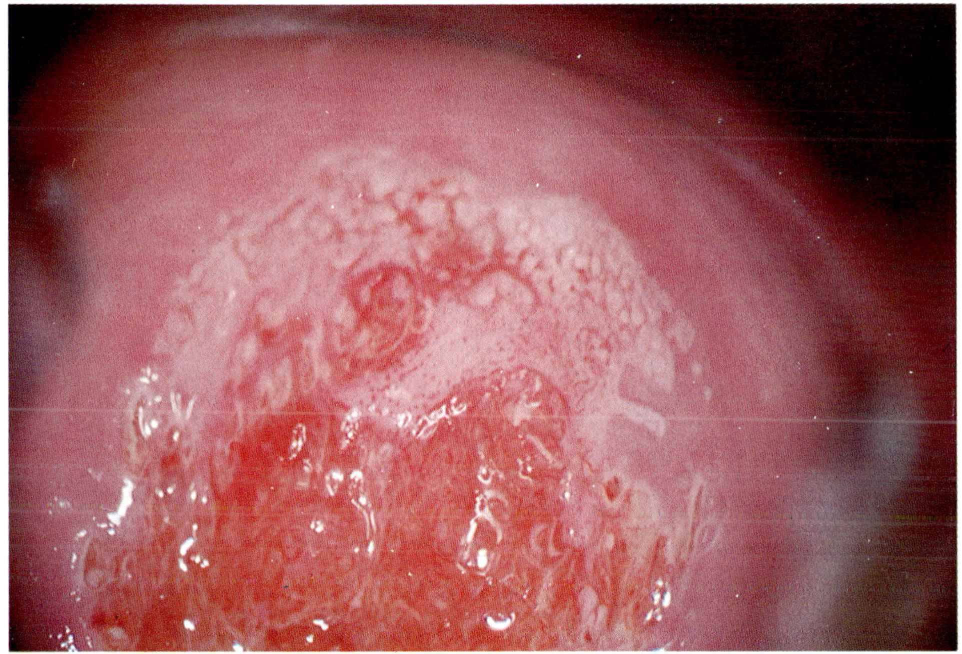

Figure 29. Colpophotograph (12.5×) of anterior lip of cervix showing an atypical transformation zone in a 22-year-old G_1AB_1 female with a two year history of repeated Class 3 cytology. Note the white epithelium with regular mosaic structure and the focus of white epithelium with delicate punctation at 12 o'clock. Biopsy of these areas revealed moderate dysplasia.

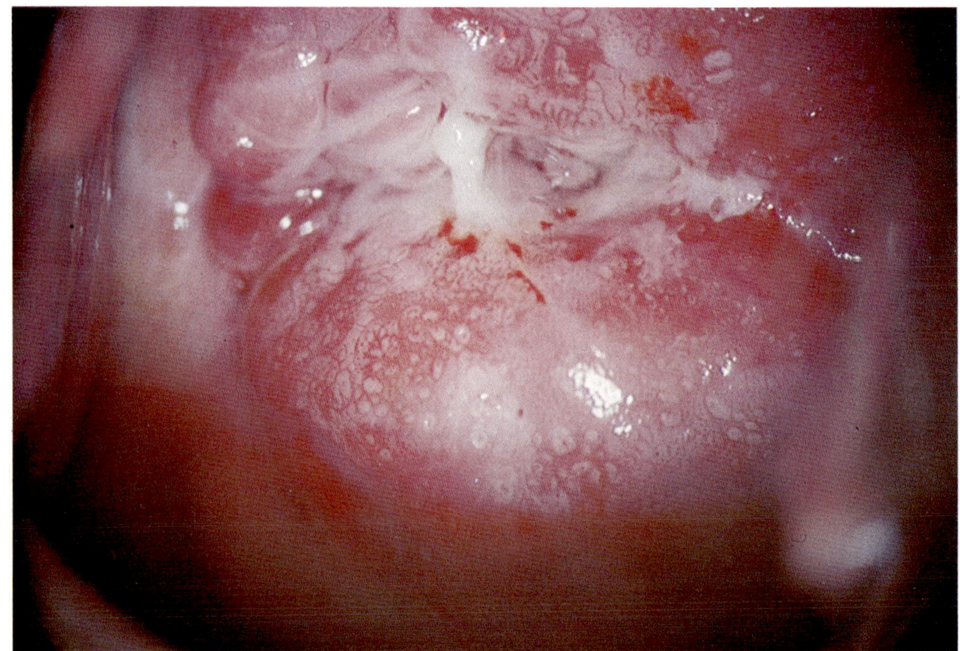

Figure 30. Colpophotograph of the cervix of a 26-year-old G_2P_2 female referred for investigation of a Class 3 Papanicolaou smear. Photo shows coarse punctation, mosaic, and reverse mosaic structure (12.5×). Biopsy of this area showed severe dysplasia with foci of carcinoma in-situ.

intercapillary distance depending upon the degree of associated histologic atypia. Punctation may be delicate and regular with normal intercapillary distance. Alternatively, capillary loops may appear markedly dilated and tortuous with increased distance between individual vessels. Mosaic terminal vessels also may be fine or coarse, and regular or irregular; such vessels may outline fields which are small, large, round, polygonal, and so forth. Increased intercapillary distance and irregularity of mosaic tiles is caused by a disordered compression and disappearance of some stromal papillae by the rapidly proliferating atypical epithelium. In general, the more irregular the mosaic pattern, the more significant is the histologic lesion. A diffuse, symmetrical mosaic pattern is more often a feature of normal metaplasia than of neoplasia. The presence of a small capillary within the center of a mosaic tile increases the significance of the mosaic pattern (Fig. 31).

Squamous metaplasia without any apparent malignant potentiality can also exhibit patterns of punctation and mosaic. The mosaic in many places consists of delicate terminal capillaries coursing around small gland openings. This is not surprising, since there is a transient period during the development of the normal transformation zone when columnar papillae appear surrounded by metaplastic tissue. There are certain characteristics which indicate that punctation and mosaic patterns are likely to be innocuous; the color of the epithelium is normal (the cells are not atypical and therefore not white and opaque), the surface is smooth and level with the adjacent original squamous epithelium, and the border of the lesion is indefinite or obscure. New capillary networks usually are seen forming within mosaic fields, making intercapillary distance essentially normal.

True punctation will generally be found only within a well demarcated area of white epithelium. Punctation, or diffuse capillary increase, without an associated white lesion, occurs in normal, atrophic, or inflammatory states and has only minor significance. Mosaic structure in the absence of white epithelium is not uncommonly seen in normal metaplasia.

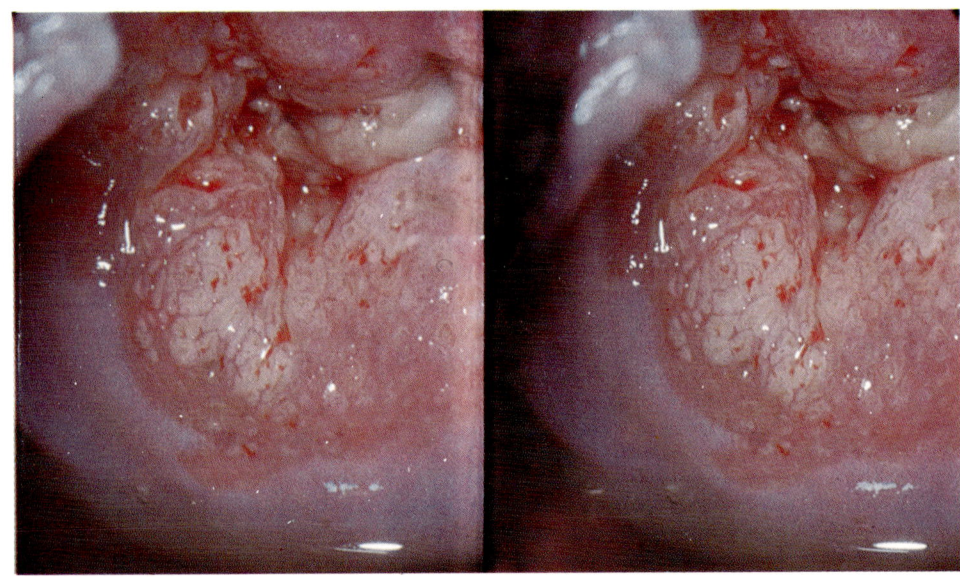

Figure 31. Leisegang stereophotograph of posterior lip of cervix of a 23-year-old G_2P_1 female with a two year history of repeated Class 3 cytology. This examination was performed at 20 weeks gestation. Photo shows an atypical transformation zone with white epithelium featuring irregular mosaic tiles encircled by coarse vessels of increased intercapillary distance (13.5×). Note the single punctation vessels within each mosaic tile, particularly at 4 to 6 o'clock position, as well as the raised and undulating surface contour. Biopsy revealed invasive carcinoma.

Mosaic and punctation vessels, in general, are characterized by a certain regularity of configuration. Their significance is related primarily to degree of vascular dilatation, intercapillary distance, and presence within areas of sharply demarcated white epithelium (Fig. 32).

KERATOSIS

Keratosis (leukoplakia), unlike other abnormalities of the transformation zone, can be diagnosed without colposcopy. It is seen prior to the application of acetic acid and without the aid of low power magnification (Fig. 33). Histologically, leukoplakia shows merely hyperkeratosis or parakeratosis (hence the new term, keratosis). Keratosis appears as a clearly demarcated, white area with an irregular border. The white appearance is due to deflection of incident light by a dense layer of superficial cornified epithelium. Usually the surface is flat but raised above the surrounding epithelium. Because of its considerable opacity, keratosis obscures the underlying vascular architecture and prevents analysis of the underlying tissue structure. Keratosis can cover areas of pathologic epithelium, albeit infrequently.

Localization of keratosis is important. When it overlies normal squamous epithelium, it usually is of no significance. When present within the transformation zone, especially when surrounded by white epithelium, mosaic, or punctation, it is obviously quite disturbing. It is sometimes instructive to remove an area of keratosis in an effort to unmask punctation and mosaic structure. Although keratosis is more often found in connection with benign lesions, the possibility of an underlying precancerous lesion or even well differentiated carcinoma must always be kept in mind. For this reason, all keratotic areas require biopsy.

ABNORMAL BLOOD VESSELS

Foci of abnormal epithelium within an atypical transformation zone may exhibit terminal vessels which lack regularity. Such capillaries are referred to as atypical vessels. They are irregular

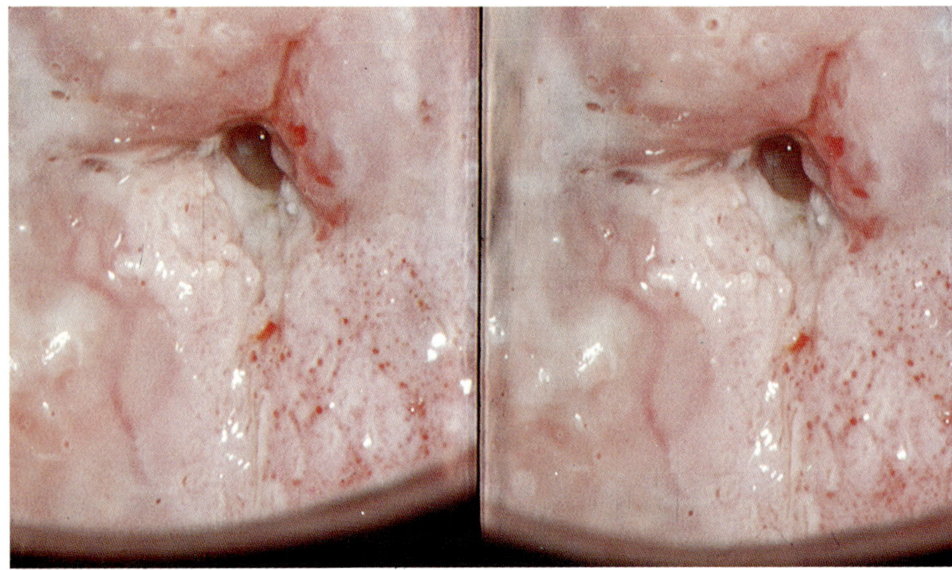

Figure 32. Leisegang stereophotograph (13.5×) of the cervix of a 51-year-old G_4P_4 female with questionable carcinoma in situ on Papanicolaou smear. Note the irregular surface contour and white epithelium with coarse punctation. Biopsy of this area revealed early invasive carcinoma.

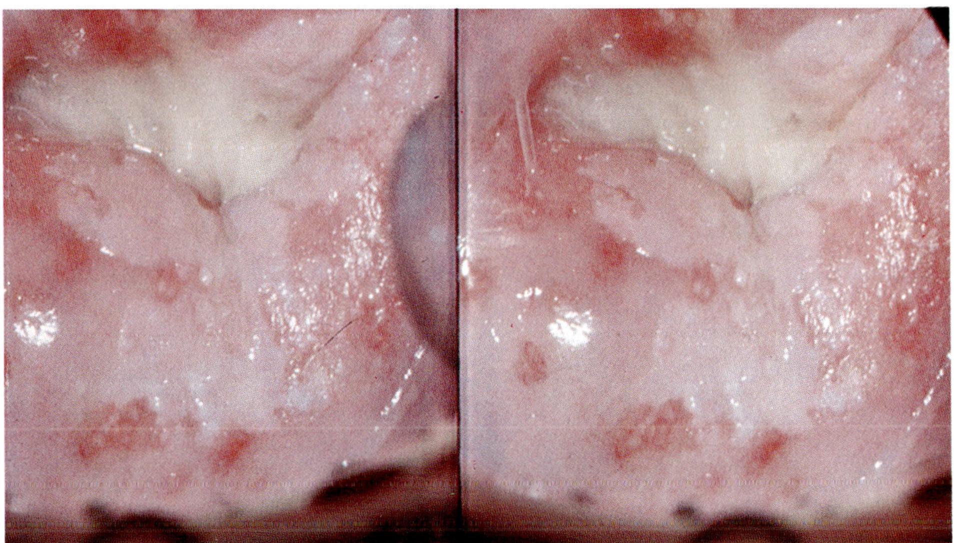

Figure 33. Leisegang stereophotograph of the cervix of a 31-year-old G_4P_3 female at 10 weeks gestation with a cervical smear suggestive of dysplasia. Photo is taken prior to application of acetic acid (13.5×). Note the raised white epithelium (keratosis) on the posterior lip. Biopsy of this area revealed moderate dysplasia. The intense white material at the cervical os is cervical mucus.

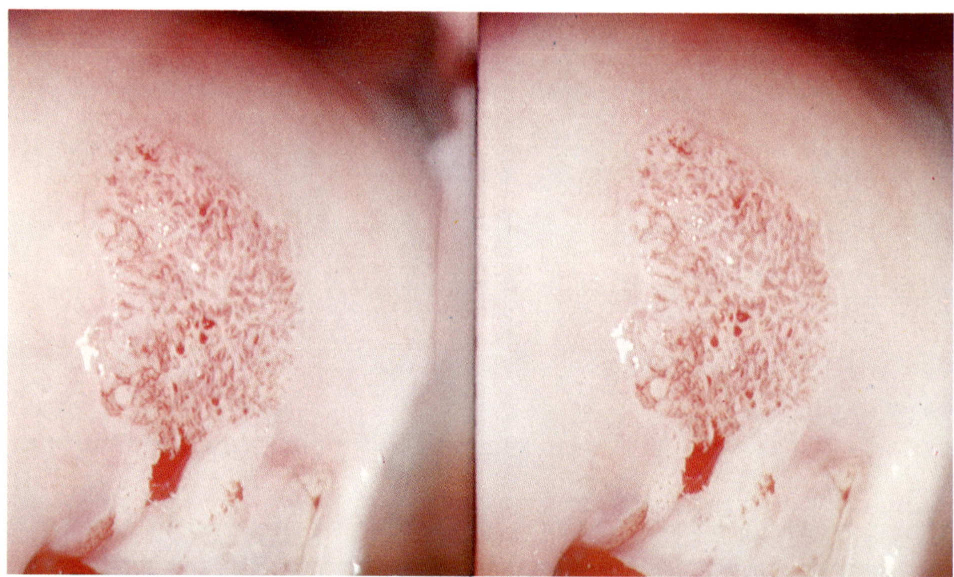

Figure 34. Leisegang stereophotograph showing an isolated group of atypical blood vessels seen after application of acetic acid to the cervix of a 51-year-old G_2P_2 female with abnormal Papanicolaou smears for two years (13.5×). Biopsy of this area revealed moderate to severe dysplasia.

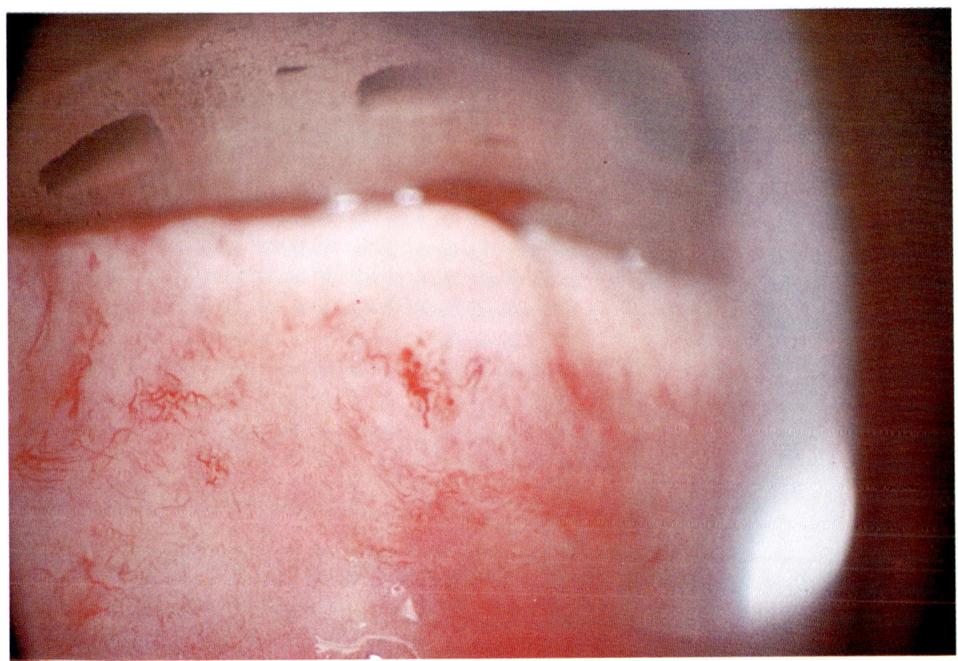

Figure 35. Colpophotograph of apex of vagina in a 47-year-old G_3P_3 female. Photo is taken three years following radiation treatment to the cervix for Stage 1 squamous cell carcinoma (20×). Note the various configurations and random distribution of abnormal blood vessels.

in contour, calibre, and mutual arrangement and frequently display a greater than normal intercapillary distance. They may appear colposcopically as a coarse meshwork enclosing irregular avascular fields, as irregularly branched patterns showing no steady decrease in diameter of terminal branches, or as single vessels with sharp, irregular bends (Figs. 34 and 35).

Table 4. Intercapillary distance and histologic diagnosis*

Histologic Diagnosis	*Intercapillary Distance >300 μ (%)*
Benign lesions	1.8
Dysplasia	14.6
Carcinoma in situ	57.1
Early invasive carcinoma	76.9
Invasive carcinoma	85.5
Normal mucous membrane of cervix = 50 to 250 μ	

*(From Kolstad, P.: Acta Obstet. Gynecol. Scand. 43(Suppl. 7):105, 1964.)

Alterations in angioarchitecture, manifested by the random distribution of coarse, coiled, and irregularly branching vessels reminiscent of commas, corkscrews, or spaghetti are correlated with the degree of malignant histologic change. Vessels of this nature are most often colposcopic indicators of carcinoma in situ or invasive disease (Table 4).

GRADING A LESION

Interpretation of the atypical transformation zone may often be aided by grading the colposcopic appearance (Table 5). Grade 1 lesions show flat white epithelium and a regular pattern of fine calibre vessels. Grade 2 lesions exhibit flat but whiter epithelium along with an irregular pattern of vessels, often coarse in quality. Grade 3 lesions display white epithelium with irregular surface contour and irregular, coarse, and coiled vessels.

Although the atypical transformation zone identifies the site and extent of major dysplastic and cancerous epithelia, many atypical transformation zones demonstrate only minor histologic disturbances in cervical epithelia and are of no apparent clinical

Table 5. Grades on atypical transformation zone*

Grade	Colposcopic Findings
1	Flat, white epithelium with or without a regular pattern of fine caliber vessels
2	Flat, white epithelium with or without an irregular pattern of coarse caliber vessels
3	Very white epithelium, with an irregular pattern of coarse caliber, coiled or bizarre branching vessels, usually wide intercapillary distance, and an irregular surface contour

Grade	Surface	Color	Capillaries
1	Flat	White	Fine
2	Flat	White	Dilated
3	Irregular	Whitest	Coiled

Grade 1 = "Abnormal" epithelium
Grade 2 = Minor dysplasia—carcinoma
Grade 3 = Carcinoma
*(From Coppleson, M., et al.: *Colposcopy: A Scientific and Practical Approach to the Cervix in Health and Disease*. Charles C Thomas, Springfield, Ill., 1971, with permission.)

significance. Therefore, colposcopic gradings often correlate with histology, but not invariably. In general, the greater the histologic abnormality, the more pronounced are the colposcopic changes. Grade 1 lesions generally correlate with "abnormal epithelium" (i.e., minor dysplasias, parakeratoses). Grade 2 lesions generally correlate with lesions varying from minor dysplasias to carcinoma in situ. Grade 3 lesions are most likely those of carcinoma in situ or preclinical invasive carcinoma.

It is possible for colposcopists with vast experience to differentiate the various forms of cervical intraepithelial neoplasia from each other and from early invasive cancer on the basis of colposcopic features alone (i.e., color, surface contour, vascularity, and grading of quality). However, gynecologists practicing clinical colposcopy should guard against the temptation to make histologic diagnoses and should remember that all keratoses, white epithelium, punctation, and mosaic structures, and areas of abnormal vasculature require biopsy for definitive confirmation of the true nature of the lesion.

7

MISCELLANEOUS COLPOSCOPIC FINDINGS

Any process of inflammation, infection, regeneration, or repair on the cervix or vagina can exhibit features which when viewed through a colposcope may resemble those of an atypical transformation zone due to neoplasia. Areas of punctation, mosaic structure, white epithelium, keratosis, and even abnormal blood vessels can be observed which are unrelated to metaplasia, either normal or atypical. Coexistent morphologic characteristics previously outlined—specifically epithelial whiteness, surface contour, vascular configuration, and sharpness or diffuseness of tissue boundaries—in most instances should clarify the nature of the above mentioned benign conditions. Clearly, if any doubt exists, a biopsy should be taken.

VAGINOCERVICITIS

Trichomonas vaginalis infestation usually creates inflammation of surface epithelium; a diffuse, hyperemic state of the squamous epithelium of the ectocervical and vaginal mucosa results. Through a colposcope Trichomonas vaginalis vaginitis is seen as generalized punctation within a relatively translucent and flat epithelial surface. The involvement of the cervix and vaginal walls is diffuse; this characteristic differentiates this lesion from punctation on a sharply demarcated white backgound which is characteristic of an atypical transformation zone. Coiling of capillaries within dermal papillae which penetrate to the tissue surface produces typical "strawberry spots" peculiar to Trichomonas vaginitis (Fig. 36).

TRUE EROSION

True erosion is a term used to define a localized absence of surface epithelium. It has occasionally been applied erroneously and inappropriately to the presence of columnar tissue on the exocervix. In the early literature "erosia vera" was considered to be indicative of neoplasia. However, it is now understood that most true erosions arise from trauma related to instrumentation. Denuding of squamous epithelium occurs most often from introduction and manipulation of vaginal specula. The thin, friable, atrophic cervical mucosa of the postmenopausal female is especially subject to such injury. Trauma is not uncommon in some atypical transformation zones, particularly when the surface is raised, irregular, or thickened. The epithelial edge is often damaged, lifted from its underlying stroma, and rolled over onto itself.

Inspection of the intact epithelium surrounding a focus of erosion will usually reveal the true nature of the lesion. Obviously, an erosion surrounded by an atypical transformation zone has greater significance than erosion encircled by normal, healthy tissue.

ATROPHIC EPITHELIUM

Upon withdrawal of endogenous estrogen during menopause, the transformation zone usually recedes out of sight into the endocervical canal. The squamous epithelium of the cervix and vagina becomes flat and thin. Individual cells shrink; their nuclei decrease in size and the ratio of nucleus to cytoplasm diminishes. Consequently, postmenopausal squamous epithelium is more permeable to light from the colposcope, and the stromal vascular pattern below the transparent epithelium is ac-

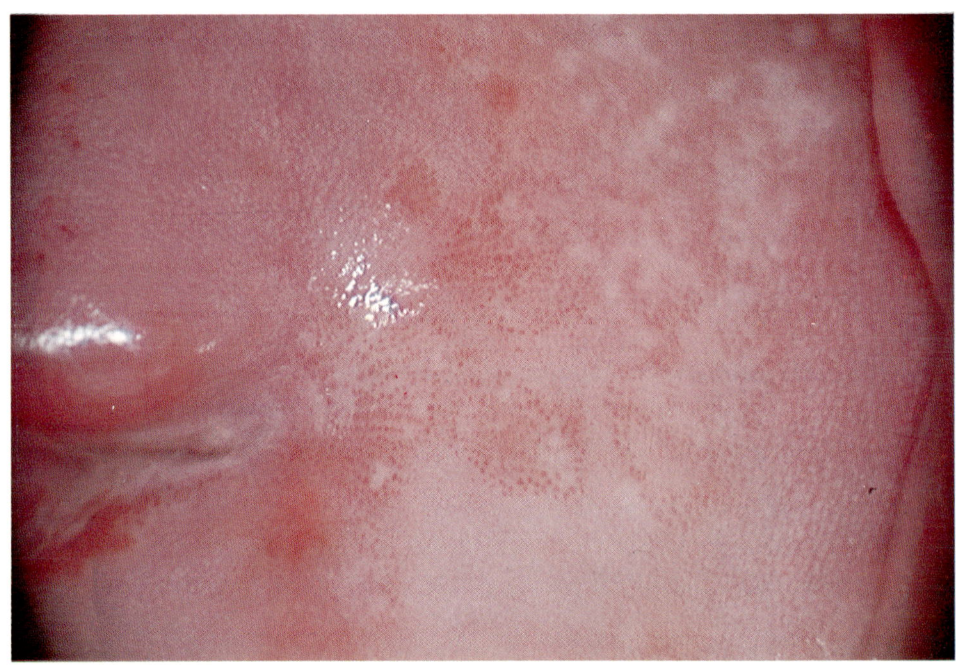

Figure 36. Colpophotograph of cervix showing diffuse punctation with "rosettes" characteristic of trichomonas, especially at 3 o'clock position (20×).

centuated. Because the stromal vessels are fragile and lie close to the tissue surface, they can be easily damaged, and small subepithelial hemorrhages may develop. The mere application of acetic acid is frequently traumatic enough to produce multiple petechiae of varying sizes.

CONDYLOMA AND PAPILLOMA

The condylomata and papillomata are exophytic lesions which can be present on the cervix both within and outside the transformation zone. They are frequently multifocal and can also be found in the vagina and on the vulva. Such lesions are of particular importance since they may constitute the source of abnormal cytology and may thus be mistaken for keratinizing cancer.

The surface of a condyloma acuminatum or papilloma is usually undulating; a complicated stromal core with numerous new vessels may be seen (Fig. 37). Often the epithelium has a white appearance prior to the application of acetic acid. If one observes a delicate array of tiny vessels in reticular formation, the benign nature of the lesion is confirmed.

CRYOSURGERY AND ELECTROCAUTERY

Colposcopic findings following cryosurgery and electrocautery are influenced by the histopathologic changes that occur as a result of local tissue destruction and repair.

Immediately after freezing, the affected tissue can be delineated from adjacent nonfrozen tissue by the presence of increased opacity and atypical vascular patterns. Approximately six hours subsequent to treatment, extensive tissue necrosis is apparent. The frozen area is covered by a membrane which has a greyish-white appearance. Twenty-four hours following injury caused by cold, intense squamous proliferation begins at the periphery of the frozen zone. This effect, when viewed through a colposcope, is characterized by the presence of white epithelium. Blood vessels are also exaggerated and assume abnormal configurations. At this time it is extremely difficult to

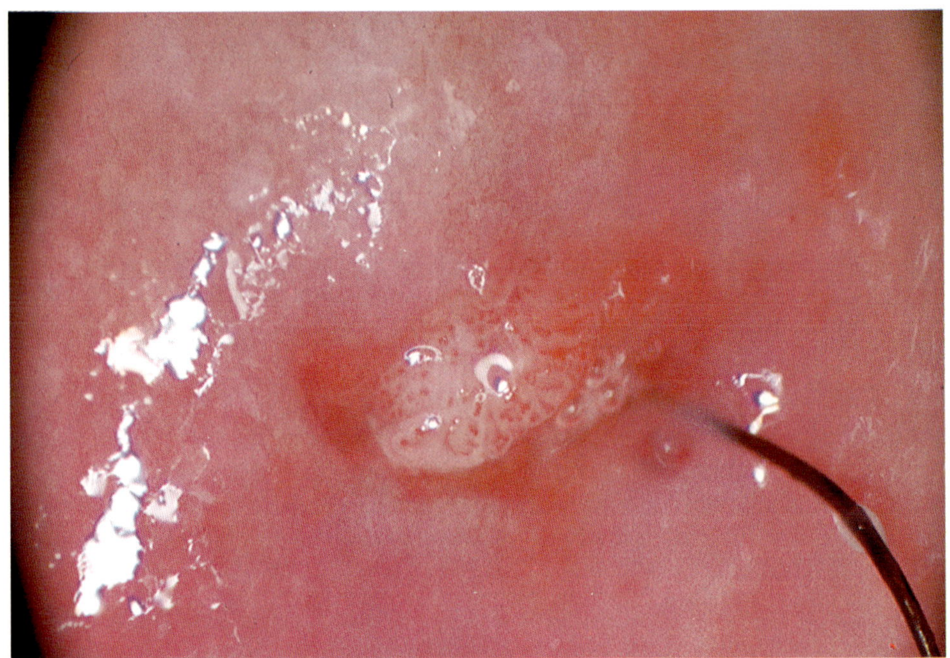

Figure 37. Colpophotograph of exocervix with papilloma extruding from cervical os (12.5×). Note the numerous blood vessels in the papilloma and the IUD string in lower right of picture.

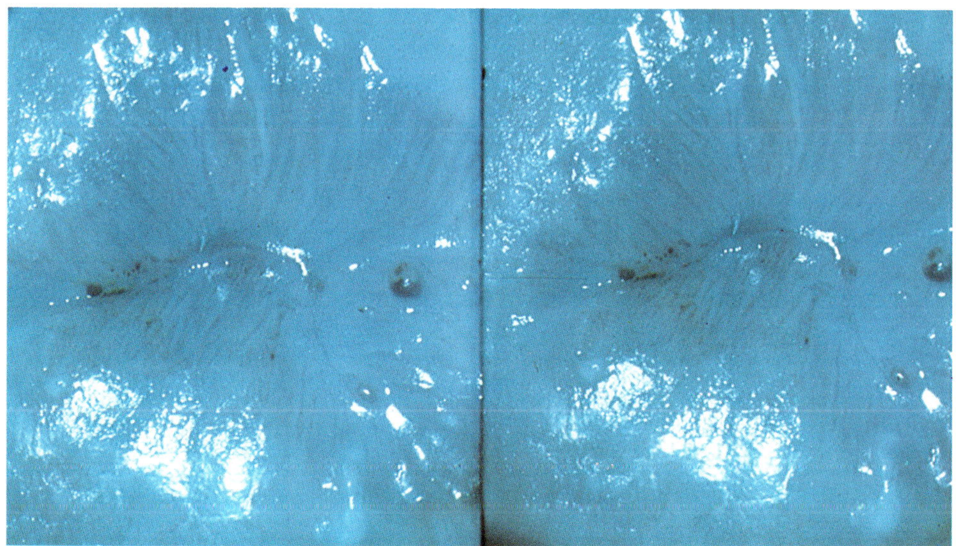

Figure 38. Leisegang stereophotograph of a cervix approximately two years post cryosurgery. Photograph is taken through a green filter (13.5×). Note the symmetrical alignment of blood vessels radiating from the external cervical os. Such vessels typify the process of regeneration.

distinguish by colposcopy the young regenerating squamous epithelium from dysplastic or even neoplastic tissue. Biopsies of suspicious areas demonstrate an intense healing response. Rarely do they reveal any neoplastic or dysplastic changes.

During the first three months following cryotherapy, a mosaic pattern with some punctation can be seen. At three to five months, punctation is the principal colposcopic finding. After one year, keratosis sometimes appears, with or without associated punctation or mosaic structure. Normality returns within 6 to 20 months, although punctation and linear vessels of regeneration may persist.

The residual colposcopic appearance long after cautery is that of smooth, translucent squamous epithelium in which streaks of delicate terminal vessels radiate centrifugally from the external os as spokes of a wheel. This ultimate index of regeneration is also seen following cryosurgery (Fig. 38).

When cryosurgery or electrocautery is employed as local treatment for cervical intraepithelial neoplasia, followup colposcopic examination should not be carried out for at least three to six months following tissue destruction. This will avoid the inevitable confusion attributable to any colposcopic features of atypia that may be present and ensure the presence of mature regenerative vascular changes.

RADIATION

Changes observable through a colposcope following exposure of the vagina to radiation are primarily those related to severely abnormal angioarchitecture. Vessels take on bizarre shapes and patterns which, by the inexperienced colposcopist, can easily be mistaken for recurrence of the initial neoplastic process (Fig. 35). Abnormal blood vessels following radiotherapy generally present themselves on a background of translucent and flat rather than white and raised epithelium. The abnormal colposcopic pattern produced by irradiation becomes fixed at an interval of approximately six months following treatment. If a change

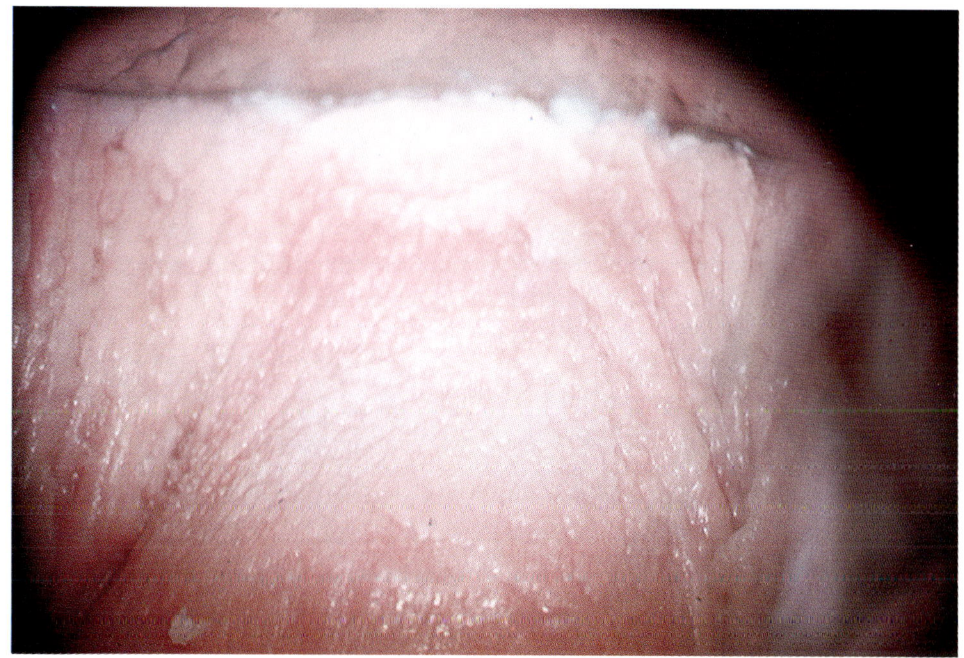

Figure 39. Colpophotograph of anterior vaginal fornix (12.5×). Note the thickened, keratinized epithelium produced by diaphragm use.

occurs in the vascular or epithelial character after six months, colposcopically directed biopsy is indicated since recurrent cancer is probable.

DIAPHRAGMS

The regular use of a diaphragm for contraception produces a characteristic colposcopic picture. Presumably as a result of continued abrasion of the squamous epithelium of the vaginal fornices, areas of acanthosis and hyperkeratosis develop. Under the colpsocope these localized areas exhibit a raised, irregular surface (Fig.39). Blood vessels are usually absent. Keratosis can be present. In general, affected tissue appears frosty rather than white and is not well circumscribed.

8

EVALUATION OF DIETHYLSTILBESTROL EXPOSED OFFSPRING

Since Herbst, Scully and others noted the association of maternal ingestion of stilbestrol during pregnancy with vaginal clear cell adenocarcinoma in the offspring, attention has focused on diagnostic and evaluative screening methods of young women at risk by virtue of intrauterine exposure. The degree of risk is not clearly defined; but in various series of women who were studied because their mothers took diethylstilbestrol (DES) during pregnancy, the offspring had vaginal adenosis in approximately 90 percent of the cases. The frequency with which vaginal adenosis is encountered in these offspring is particularly worrisome because adenosis is so often found to coexist in or about foci of adenocarcinoma. Until the exact relation between vaginal adenosis and the subsequent development of vaginal malignancy (clear cell adenocarcinoma or stratified squamous carcinoma) has been determined by long term study, all women whose mothers ingested stilbestrol during pregnancy must be followed.

Colposcopy has now been shown to be an excellent method for screening, for specifying the biopsy sites, and for following both the extent and possible progression of the vaginal and cervical lesions.

Both on gross inspection and with the colposcope one can

detect the presence of non-neoplastic conditions in the genital tract now recognized to be due to in utero exposure to DES. These fall into two general categories: (1) the red cervix, also called congenital erosion, ectopy, or erythroplakia, in which the cervix has a grossly red appearance. With the colposcope, prior to the application of acetic acid, this coloration is seen to be due to the numerous normal appearing blood vessels in the submucosa. With the application of acetic acid the area involved is covered with the grapes of columnar epithelium similar to that seen in the original native columnar epithelium of the endocervix. Not infrequently some of the grapes are enlarged to sizes rarely seen except in adenosis (Fig. 40). (2) Vaginal and cervical ridges (hood, cockscomb, pseudopolyp formation). The hood is a fold of mucous membrane surrounding the portio of the cervix (Fig. 41). It very often disappears if the portio is pulled down with a tenaculum or displaced with a speculum. The cockscomb is an atypical appearance of the anterior lip of the cervix which is peaked (Fig. 42). Vaginal ridges are protruding circumferential bands in the upper vagina which may hide the cervix (Fig.43). Pseudopolyp formation occurs when the portio of the cervix is rather small and protrudes through a wide cervical hood (Fig. 44). When one sees any of these non-neoplastic gross stigmata, the probability that adenosis will be present is about 95 percent.

When these patients are subjected to colposcopic examination and acetic acid is applied to the cervix and vagina one of three colposcopic lesions will develop. The first is a white epithelium usually with sharply delineated areas on the vaginal wall. Frequently, this white area extends in a triangular fashion cephalad and it may involve the posterior fornix as well. The white epithelium will often have distinct punctation within the area involved (Fig. 45). A second lesion suggests a mosaic pattern. This is usually seen on the hood as well as on the anterior fornix of the vagina (Figs. 46 and 47). Both the white epithelium and the mosaic structure may also be encountered in the lateral

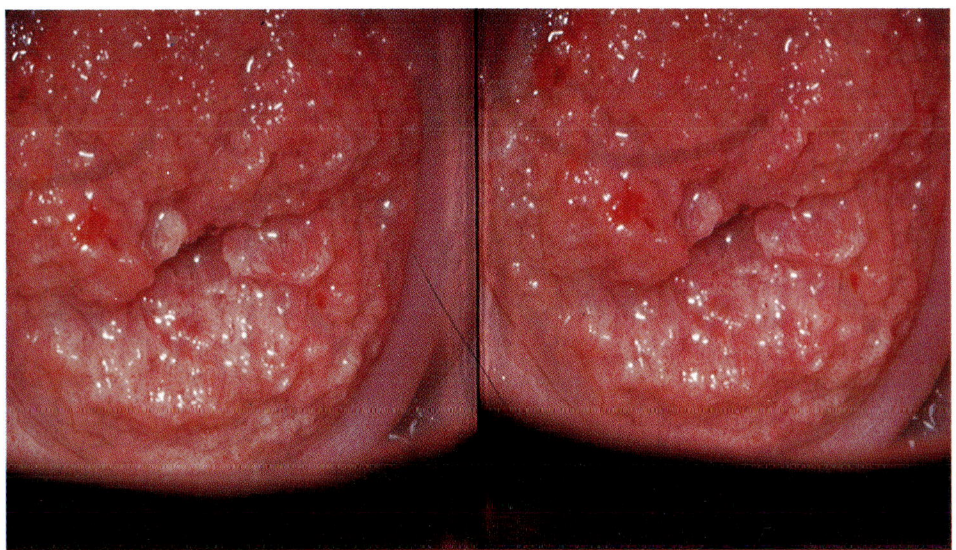

Figure 40. Leisegang stereophotograph of cervix from a patient with vaginal adenosis (13.5×). Note irregular large grapes of columnar epithelium over the entire portio of the cervix following application of acetic acid.

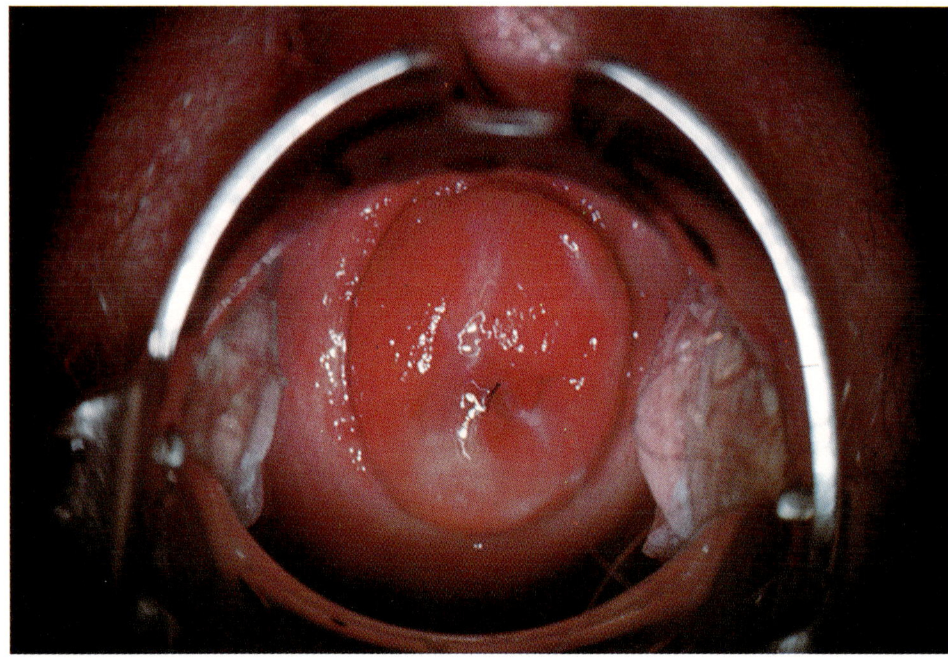

Figure 41. Colpophotograph of vaginal adenosis prior to application of acetic acid (12.5×). Columnar epithelium is present over the entire portio of the cervix (red cervix). Note that the cervical portio is completely surrounded by a hood.

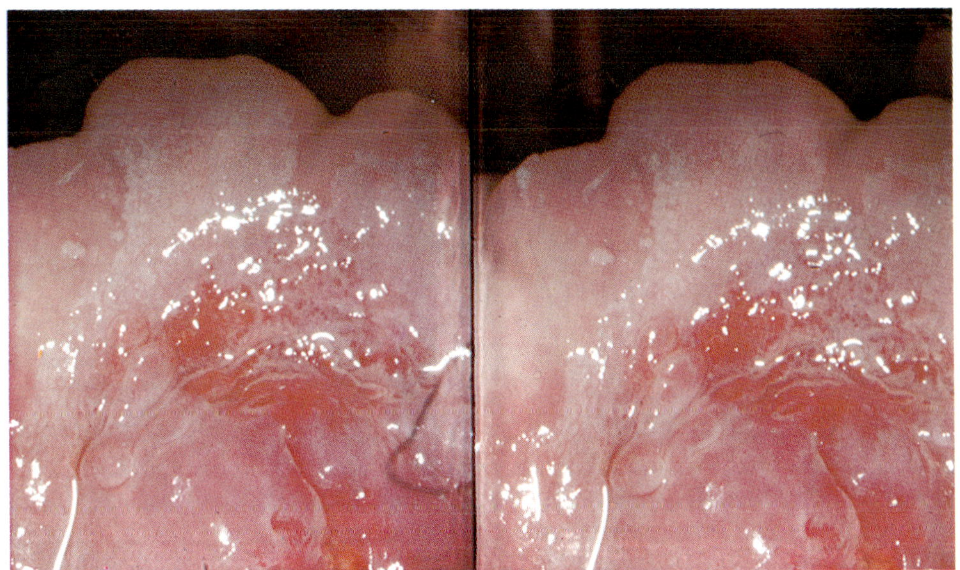

Figure 42. Leisegang colpophotograph of vaginal adenosis showing cockscomb formation of the hood (13.5×). Note the white epithelium on the hood and the metaplastic process on the portio of the cervix following the application of 3% acetic acid solution.

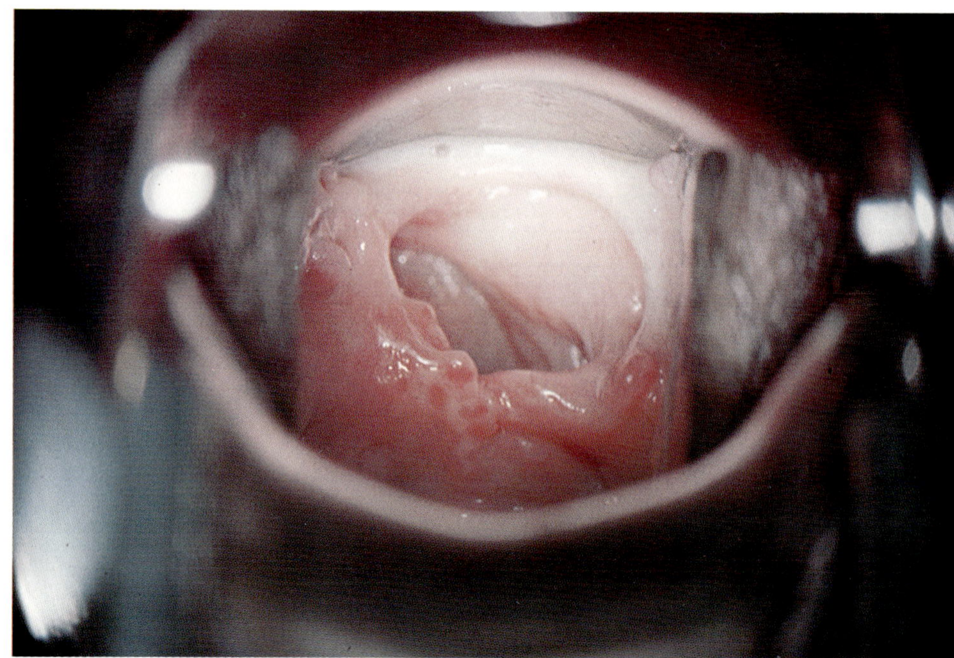

Figure 43. Colpophotograph of vaginal adenosis demonstrating a circumferential septum of the vagina (12.5×). The cervix can be seen in the distance behind the fold.

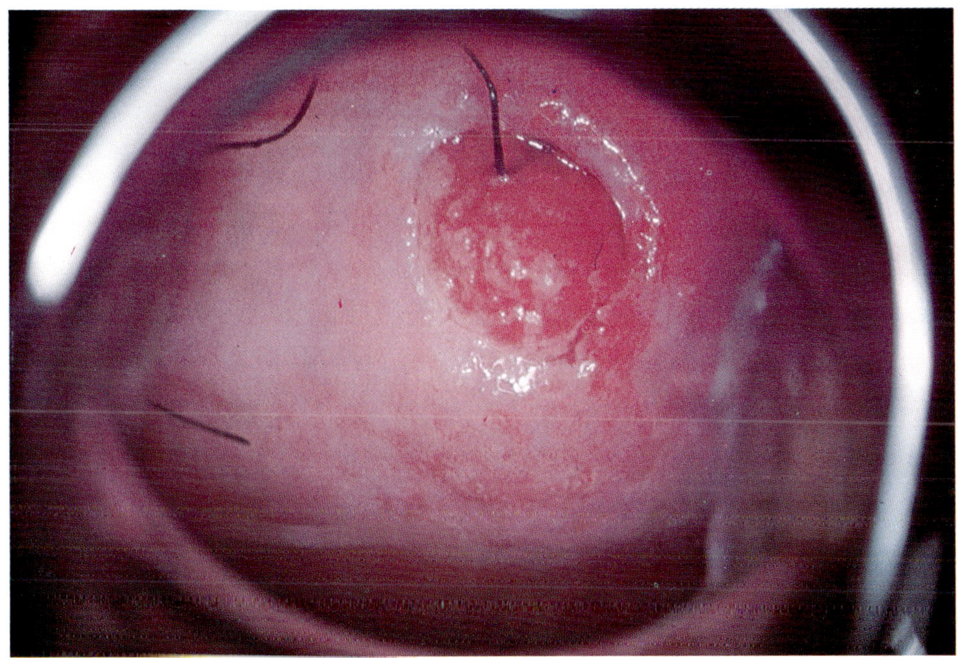

Figure 44. Colpophotograph showing a pseudopolyp of the cervix in a patient with adenosis (12.5×). Note the IUD string emanating from the os of the small portio of cervix which is covered by columnar epithelium.

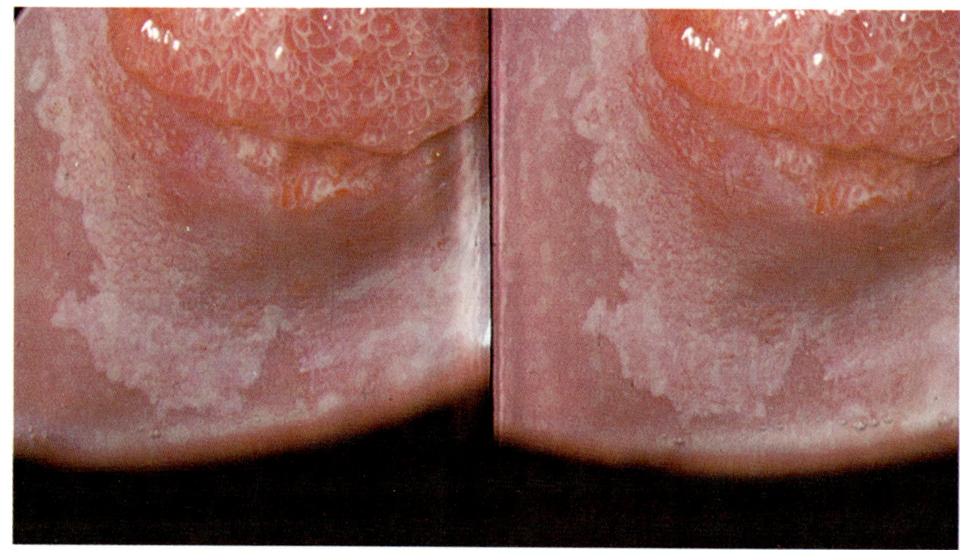

Figure 45. Leisegang colpophotograph of vaginal adenosis demonstrating white epithelium with punctation extending into the posterior vaginal fornix (13.5×). Note the grapes of columnar epithelium on the portio of the cervix. (From Obstet Gynecol 44: 259, 1974, Fig. 1B, with permission.)

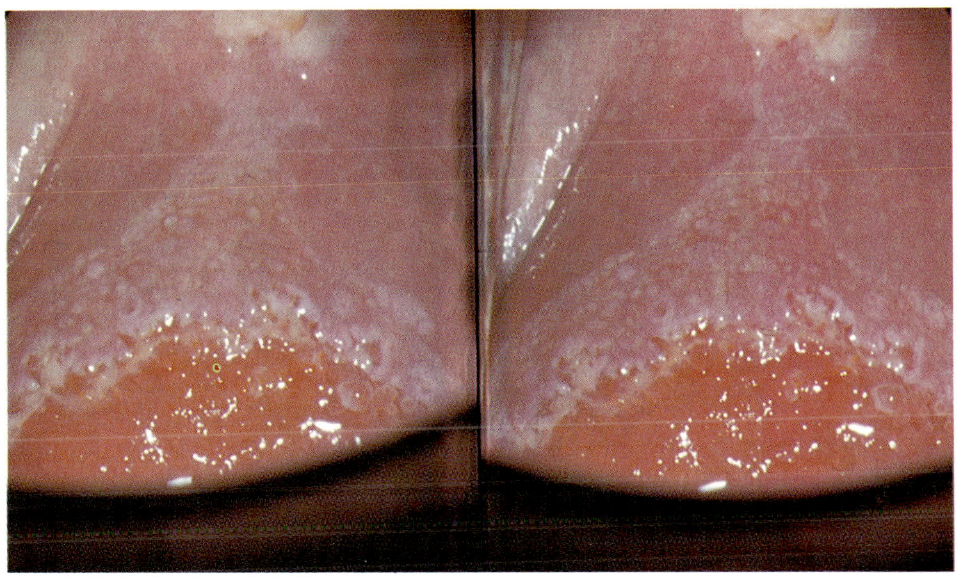

Figure 46. Leisegang colpophotograph of vaginal adenosis showing mosaic formation in the anterior fornix of the vagina (13.5×). Note the characteristic triangular distribution frequently observed. (From Obstet Gynecol 44: 259, 1974, Fig. 1B, with permission.)

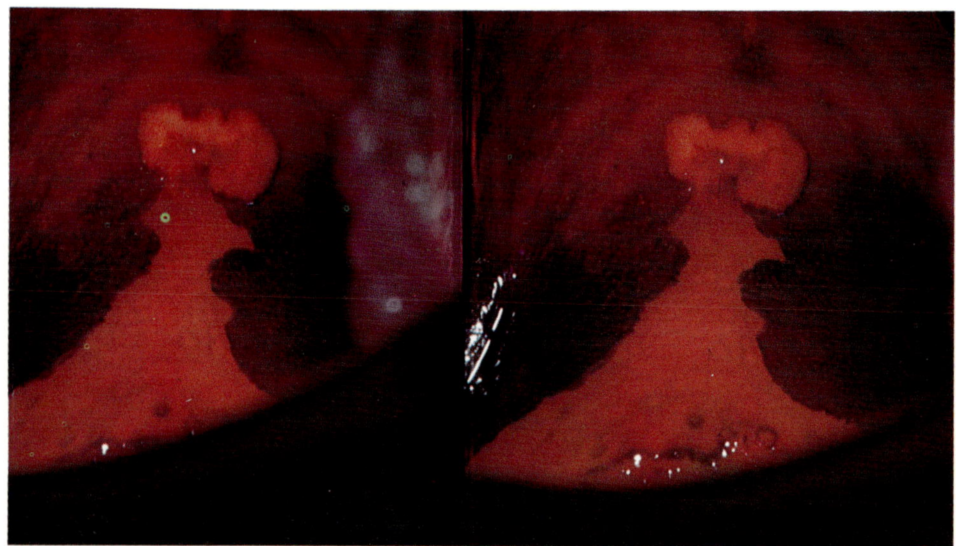

Figure 47. Leisegang colpophotograph of the same patient following application of Lugol's iodine (13.5×). Note that the area of involvement generally does not take up the stain.

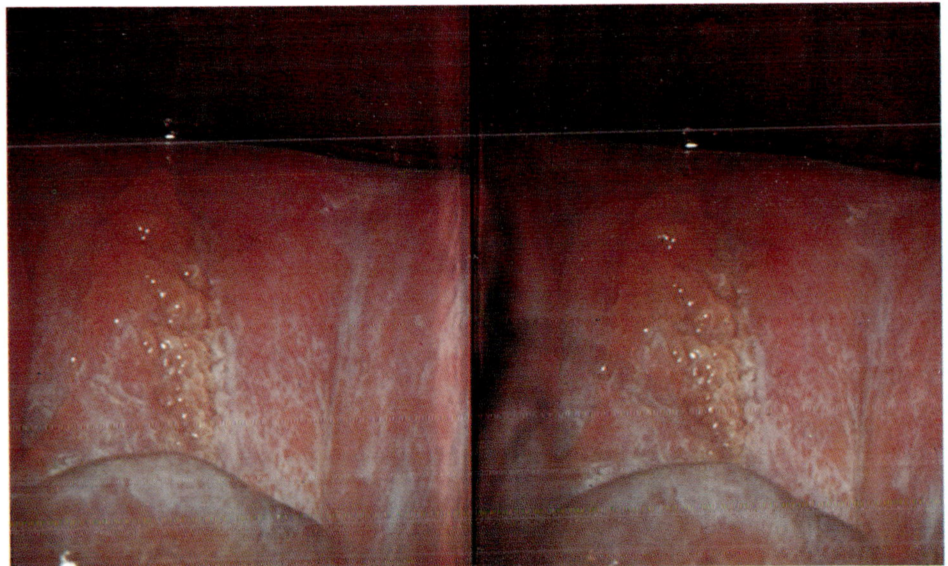

Figure 48. Leisegang colpophotograph of vaginal adenosis showing columnar epithelium involving the anterior fornix of the vagina (13.5×). Note the similarity of this tissue to the columnar epithelium on the portio of the cervix. There is white epithelium with punctation to the left of the columnar epithelium on the vaginal fornix.

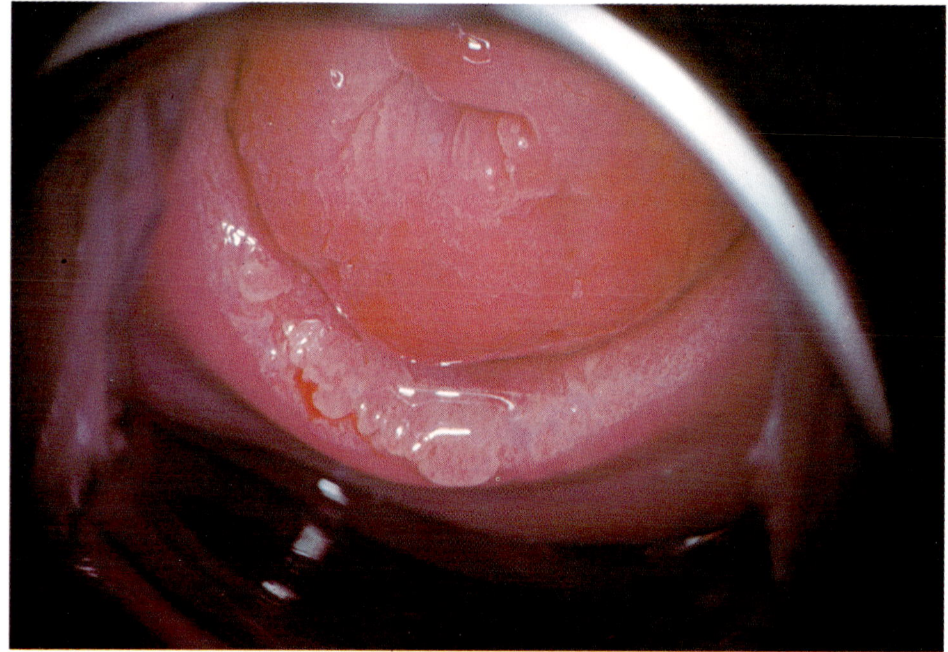

Figure 49. Colpophotograph of adenosis showing cervix covered by columnar epithelium (12.5×). Note columnar epithelium as well as white epithelium on the hood, posterior to the cervix.

fornices usually contiguous with the anterior triangular area of involvement. A third type of lesion consists of columnar epithelium whose grape-like appearance is similar to that seen in the endocervix (Figs. 48 and 49). This type of epithelium is most apt to be located in the posterior or anterolateral fornices high in the vagina.

Vaginal adenosis is characterized colposcopically by its multiplicity of appearances. The most frequent colposcopic patterns are white lesion only, mosaic only, and white and mosaic concurrently in different areas of the vagina and /or hood. One of these three patterns occurs in almost two thirds of the patients. Columnar epithelium alone is quite rare, being present in less than 5 percent of the patients.

Although most vaginal adenosis occurs in the fornices around the vagina, it is important that the mucous membrane of the entire vaginal canal be examined down to the hymenal ring. Circumferential bands may be found especially in the junction of the upper and middle thirds of the vagina. Occasionally, areas of vaginal adenosis are also seen in isolated locations along the side walls of the vagina.

Biopsies of these areas are best taken with the Eppendorfer biopsy punch. No anesthesia is necessary and the discomfort is minimal. However, if the patient is apprehensive or extremely young, one may apply either cetacaine or lidocaine in the form of a spray or gel as topical anesthesia. Sometimes one may have to tent the mucous membrane in the area of the lateral vaginal wall or in the fornices with an iris hook to enable the biopsy forceps to take purchase on the specimen. Bleeding is controlled by the application of Monsel's solution. As on the cervix, the areas of greatest colposcopic change are the areas that require biopsy.

9

EXAMINATION OF THE VULVA

In contrast to colposcopy of the vagina and cervix, colposcopy of the vulva has not been demonstrated to be a very rewarding tool for routine screening or diagnosis. Because of the thickness and density of cornified squamous epithelium of the vulva, vascular changes which take place within the underlying stroma may not be readily apparent at the tissue surface. Prolonged application of 3 percent acetic acid (for a minimum of 5 minutes) will often bring out tissue changes which indicate the true nature of the histopathology. However, alterations of color, opacity, surface contour, and vascular configuration produced by acetic acid are much less specific and less consistent for lesions of the vulva than for lesions of the cervix or vagina.

Colposcopy of the vulva is generally impractical unless a gross lesion is clearly evident there. Once a lesion has been identified, colposcopy provides a valuable adjunctive technique for examination. In particular, colposcopy can determine the extent of a given lesion and allow one to investigate the presence or absence of associated vaginal involvement. Additionally, it can facilitate ascertaining the limits of tumor extension in order to define the lines of excision for adequate surgical margins. When abnormal blood vessels are observed, colposcopy of the

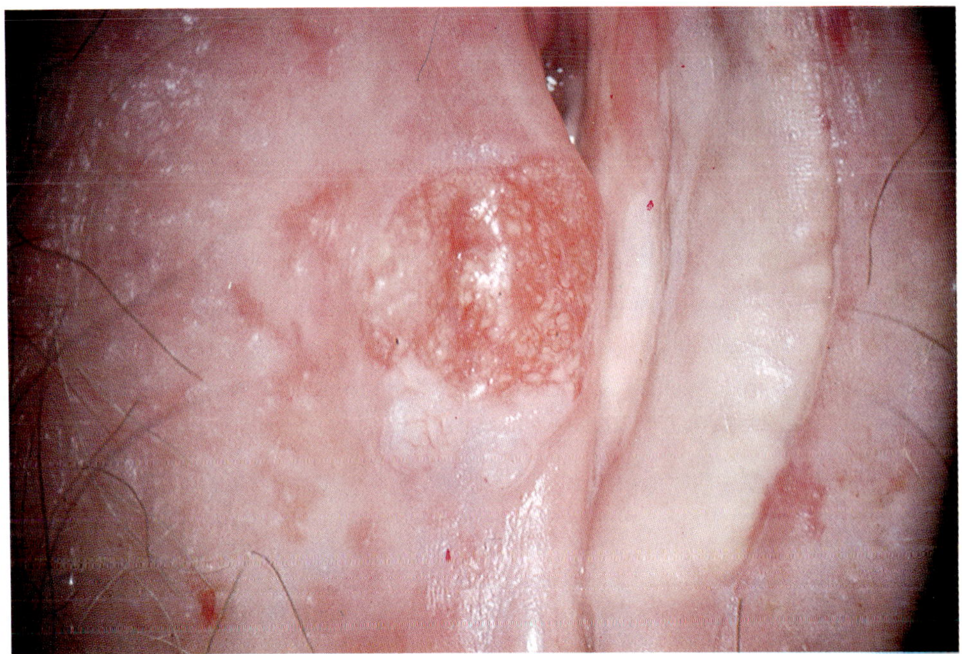

Figure 50. Colpophotograph of invasive carcinoma on the right labium minus of a 68-year-old multipara with a ten year history of vulvar pruritis (12.5×). Note the abnormal blood vessels in the areas surrounded by keratosis.

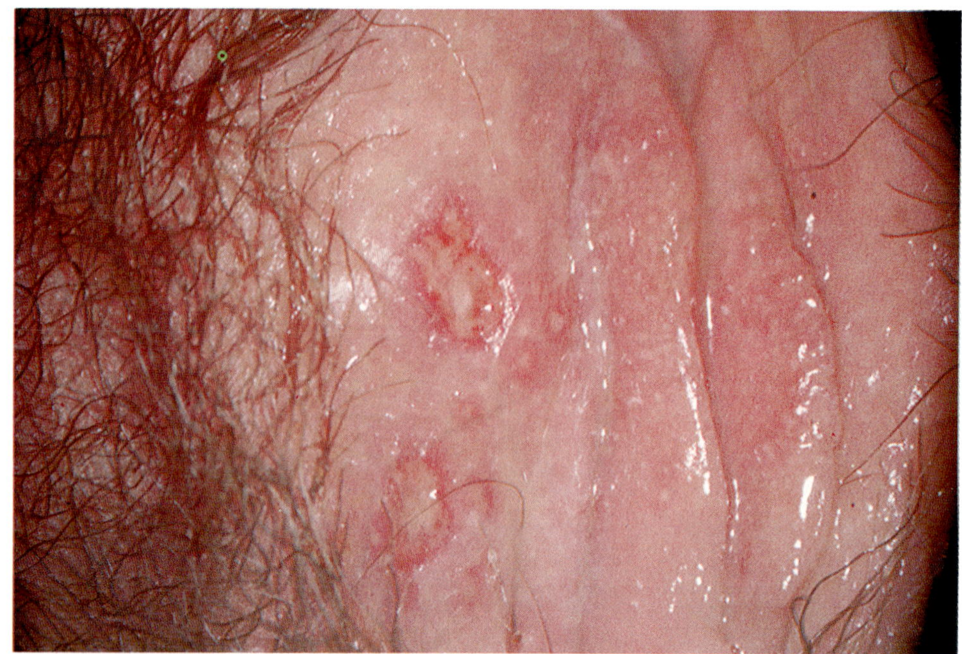

Figure 51. Colpophotograph of herpes progenitalis lesions of the vulva (8×). Note two ulcers on the medial aspect of the right labium majus. Two early satellite lesions are evident to the left of the large posterior lesion.

vulva can help one locate the most abnormal areas for purposes of directed biopsy (Fig. 50).

The basic diagnostic criteria already outlined for evaluation of the cervix can also be applied to examination of vulvar lesions. The most frequent colposcopic pattern is that of white epithelium. If a lesion is covered by keratin, the vascular pattern will not be seen colposcopically. Since it is often difficult to remove the keratin layer to expose the underlying vessels, such keratotic lesions must be excised entirely to provide an adequate biopsy. Punctation and mosaic structure are morphologic changes related to metaplasia. They are uncommon in vulvar lesions because the epithelium is thick and metaplasia is absent. The presence of atypical blood vessels within a vulvar lesion is the best indicator of malignant disease. Many benign conditions, such as herpes progenitalis ulcers, have no specific colposcopic diagnostic features. However, the colposcope does at least provide the magnification necessary to detect such lesions early (Fig. 51).

In cases in which neoplasm is suspected, a supravital dye—specifically a 1% aqueous solution of toluidine blue—has been advocated for use in combination with colposcopy. Because this is a nuclear stain, the intensity of the stain is directly proportional to the amount of nuclear material per unit of epithelium. Dye is applied, permitted to dry for two minutes, and is then washed with 1% acetic acid. This staining technique is nonspecific, however, and areas of inflammation or of neoplasia may take up the stain.

10

COLPOPHOTOGRAPHY AND OTHER AIDS TO COLPOSCOPY

Colpophotography is a desirable adjunct to colposcopy. In clinical practice, colpophotographs are useful especially for precise case recording, serial followup and comparison of lesions, and consultative reports. Additionally, they serve demonstration and teaching purposes; they also provide detailed material for publication and research.

All colposcopes, with the exception of the most inexpensive models, are equipped for the attachment of various kinds of photographic accessories. The Leisegang and Berkeley colposcopes produce stereoscopic transparencies for use through a special hand viewer. When stereoscopic pictures are projected on a screen, however, the three dimensional effect is lost and two adjacent 35 mm images are displayed (Fig. 21). Both Leisegang and Berkeley instruments employ a 35 mm camera body attached to the optical head and integrated into the optical system of the colposcope (Fig. 4). The camera is focused through a separate set of optics which are parallel to the viewing optics. As a consequence, one can photograph exactly what one sees. A unique, built in, "Sign-o-mat" feature makes it possible to incorporate the patient's identification onto the bottom of each slide.

The photo flash of the Leisegang colposcope consists of a high intensity electronic flash (6500 degrees K for 1/800 seconds) synchronized to shutter speed. The path of the electronic flash is the same as that of the standard viewing path. It is important that the field photographed be adequately illuminated to ensure suitable flash exposure. Highlights can be minimized by manipulation of stainless steel vaginal specula to decrease reflection or by use of specula with matte or Teflon finish.

In order to reproduce vascular patterns with the built in green light of the colposcope, a special filter must be interposed between the flash beam and the object of interest. This procedure can be somewhat awkward during the course of the colposcopic examination. The neutral density and green photographic filters are arranged in a small aluminum carrier which must be removed, rotated 180 degrees, and then replaced to provide proper color exposure.

The Leisegang colposcope is equipped with three photo lens covers. The middle sized cover should be used for regular photographs when film of an ASA rating of 100 is used. When photographs are taken with the green light, the photo objectives must not be covered. If Kodak high speed Ektachrome daylight film (ASA 160) is used, the cover with the smallest opening is required for regular color photographs and the cover with the largest opening is needed for green filter pictures. In all cases, a series of test pictures should be taken in order to determine the special characteristics of the specific instrument being used. The Leisegang photographs reproduced in this publication were obtained with Fujichrome film (ASA 100).

Photography with the Zeiss colposcope is much more complicated than with the Leisegang instrument. Two types of photographic equipment are available. With the first type, photography is carried out in the direction of the field of observation but without utilizing the lenses of the colposcope. This feature has the advantage of permitting the optical relation for colposcopy and photography to be selected independently of one another.

Thus observation and examination are not interrupted when photographs are taken.

The photographic apparatus consists of a basic body which is fixed to the colposcope by a special mount that ensures correct adjustment. One side of the basic body is connected to a camera by an intermediary piece while the other side accommodates the interchangeable lenses. The image scale of each lens is predetermined. The lenses are adjusted to the object plane of the colposcope and the plane of the film; the photographic unit is focused with the plane of the viewing optics.

The optical system of this first type of photographic unit permits light coming from the object of photographic interest to be deflected by the lens prism. The light beam penetrates the iris diaphragm and the photographic objective. The light is again deflected by the deflection mirror and exits parallel to its original pathway via the intermediate lens where the image of the object is finally formed. Since the prism situated in front of the main lens stands symmetrically between the two lens apertures of the colposcope, the axis of the photographic system runs symmetrically between the two optical axes of the observation system. This system can be used only with a long binocular tube, f = 160 mm, and objectives f = 125 and f = 200 mm. The authors have had no experience using the above system.

The alternative and more common photographic system photographs through the colposcope. To accomplish this, the light beam from the object viewed is split by an attachment called a beam splitter (Figs. 6 and 52). The splitting of the beam takes place in a light path parallel to and between the magnification changer and the binocular observation tube. Approximately one-half of the light from each of two observation beams (one for the right and one for the left eye) is deflected at right angles. A unit called a photographic adapter, attached to the beam splitter, contains a photographic lens which focuses the parallel rays in its focal plane, where the photographic film is located. It also houses a mirror producing an upright and unreversed image.

The photographic adapter accepts a special 35 mm camera body with a focal plane shutter (as well as other 35 mm or

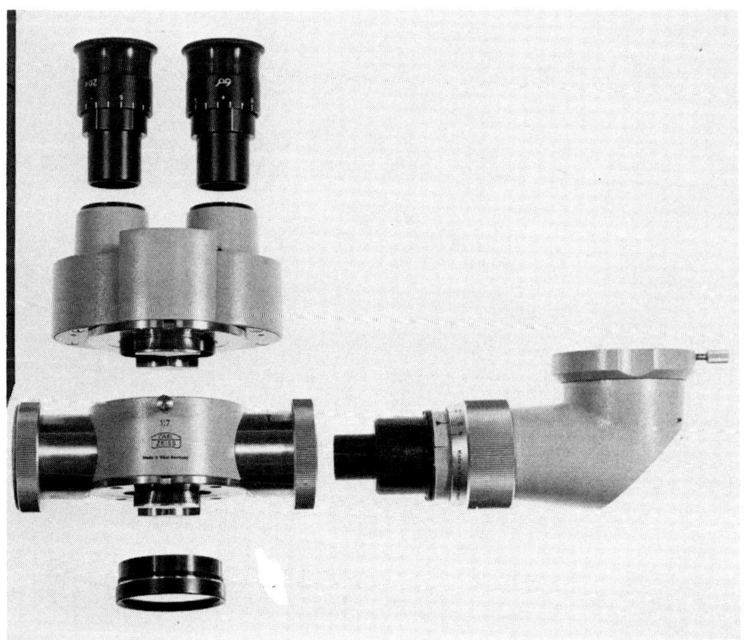

Figure 52. Photographic adapter to be attached to beam splitter.

Polaroid cameras) by interposing an appropriate intermediate ring (Fig. 53).

The photographic adapter is designed for an image field of 22 mm in diameter. This circular image reproduces the object field as it is seen using a 12.5× eyepiece regardless of which microscopic objective and setting of the magnification changer are used. Through the 20× eyepiece, the observer sees a smaller field of view at higher magnification. Since the size of the image on the film is independent of eyepiece magnification, a larger field is photographed than is actually seen through the eyepiece.

Photographs may be obtained with light from a 6 volt incandescent lamp. The setting of the microscope light must be in the high position. With an objective of 200 mm focal length, and with

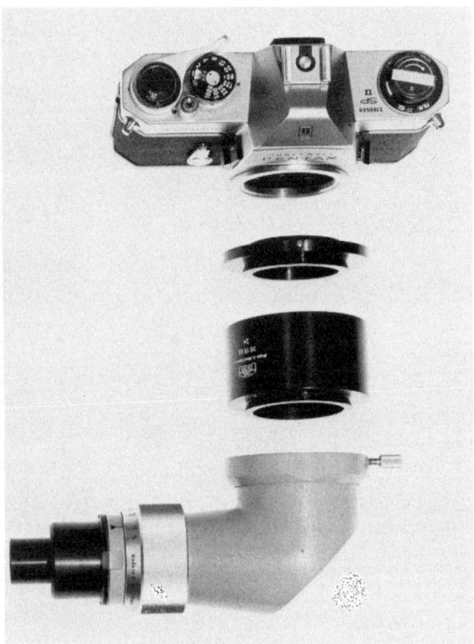

Figure 53. Intermediate ring is shown for attachment of Pentax camera.

the reversal type of color film (such as high speed Ektachrome Type B for artificial light) and an ASA rating of 125 (22 DIN), the diaphragm settings of the camera attachment would be as shown in Table 6 for the various Galilean changer settings on the colposcope.

An electronic flash illuminator is available. The power supply is usually fixed on the stand column. A plate with a dovetail groove at the bottom of the microscope body serves to hold the

Table 6. Camera diaphragm settings for Galilean changer settings

	Galilean Changer Setting				
Exposure Time	6	10	16	25	40
	Diaphragm Aperture Setting				
1/10 sec.	32	32	27	22	—
1/5 sec.	44	44	38	32	—
1/2 sec.	64	64	50	44	14

Objective: f = 200 mm
Lighting: Incandescent bulb 6V 50W/100 Overload
Reversal color film for artificial light (ASA 125)

flash illuminator. With the camera set for flash, the diaphragm opening will vary with the Galilean magnification changer settings. For 200, 250, and 300 mm objectives and daylight film (such as Fujichrome) with an ASA rating of 100 (20 DIN), the various combinations necessary to obtain adequate pictures are shown in Table 7.

Table 7. Galilean magnification setting and diaphragm opening combinations

Galilean Magnification Setting	*Diaphragm Opening*
6	32
10	32
16	22
25	16
40	14

Objective: f = 200, 250, 300 mm
Lighting: Electronic flash
Reversal type color film, daylight (ASA 100)

Since the photographic and colposcopic optics are independent elements, examinations utilizing the green filter are not photographed in green. In order to reproduce on film examinations performed with the built in green filter, the electronic flash must be covered with green material. This can be accomplished by placing a light green filter material (generally plastic) over the unit when pictures are taken. The largest diaphragm opening (f = 14) should be used.

MOTOR DRIVE

A foot pedal motor attachment for the colposcope camera is extremely helpful when several photographs are to be taken in succession. This attachment frees one's hands for focusing or performing operative procedures while the camera is being used.

OBSERVATION TUBES

Monocular observation tubes are useful for teaching purposes and are available for attachment to many different colposcopes. The authors have had experience only with those of the Leisegang and Zeiss instruments.

The Leisegang teaching tube can be used only with Leisegang camera colposcope models IL and IIIB. The tube must be placed in the same aperture in which the camera is to be inserted. Consequently, photographs cannot be taken when the teaching tube is being used.

The technique for using the teaching apparatus requires that the seated colposcopist focus the colposcope sharply on a small object in the field of view. The observer using the teaching tube must turn the ocular of the tube so that the object is clear and sharp when seen through the tube. Once this is accomplished the student's field should always be in focus along with that of the seated colposcopist; subsequent adjustment of the teaching tube should be unnecessary.

The viewing fields of instructor and student are identical; however, the field seen through the teaching tube is a mirror image of that noted by the seated viewer. The R in the teaching tube corresponds to the right side (3 o'clock) of the seated viewer's field. The L corresponds to 9 o'clock horizontal. Above the R-L horizontal is the top of the seated colposcopist's field (Fig. 54).

A focusing grid or circle can be used to measure lesions. The diameter of the center circle is 1 mm. The diameter of the largest circle is 5 mm (Fig. 54).

Since the objective lens of the teaching tube is smaller than the regular viewing objective, it is necessary to increase the light intensity to permit adequate visualization by the student observer. The photo lens cover should be removed from the photo

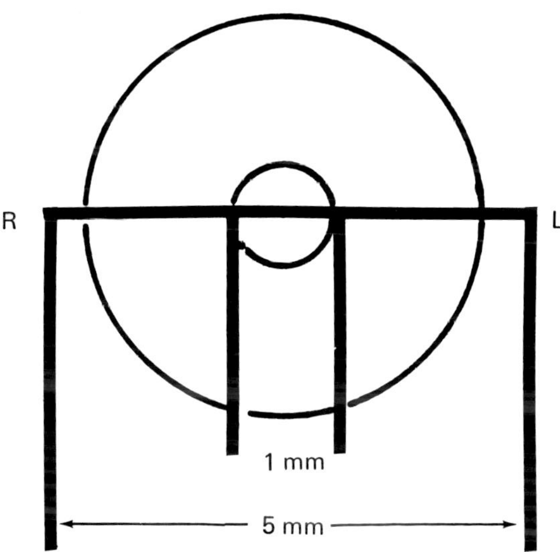

Figure 54. Area meter diagram of Leisegang colposcope observation tube.

objectives. The metal button above the rheostat knob on the transformer case should be depressed and at the same time the knob rotated clockwise. This overloads the bulb, however; therefore it should be limited to brief periods of time to avoid premature bulb burnout. The photo lens cover must be replaced when the camera is reinserted, otherwise photographs will be overexposed.

There are two observation tubes made for the Zeiss colposcope—a short tube and a long tube. The long tube is used primarily for teaching in situations where the second observer must be out of the way of a sterile field. The short tube enables the second observer to participate as an assistant in any operative use of the colposcope such as cervical conization or vaginal biopsies.

Both types of observer tubes must be used with the smaller (50) beam splitter. The tube can be attached to either the right or left of the colposcopic head and may be used in combination with either camera equipment or a second teaching tube. The teaching tubes can be pivoted about their horizontal axis of rotaion by means of a rotary prism operated by a knurled sleeve. Thus the image seen through the tube is upright and unreversed. The tube is fitted with an objective of 160 mm focal length. Magnification, field diameter, and image brightness are the same for the operator and the second observer at any position of the Galilean magnification changer provided the monocular eyepiece of the observation tube is equipped with the same eyepiece magnification as the binocular tube of the operator (Fig. 55).

CINEMATOGRAPHY

Provided the Zeiss colposcope has a beam splitter and a 6V 50W filament lamp, movies are easy to obtain. Both 16 mm and Super 8 Beaulieu cinecameras are available. A cine adapter is connected to the beam splitter. The camera is connected to the f=74 cine adapter with a C-threaded ring. The cine adapter contains a diaphragm setting motor. Via the microscope, beam splitter, and cine adapter, the light reaches a photoconductive cell in the camera. This photoconductive cell controls the motor which

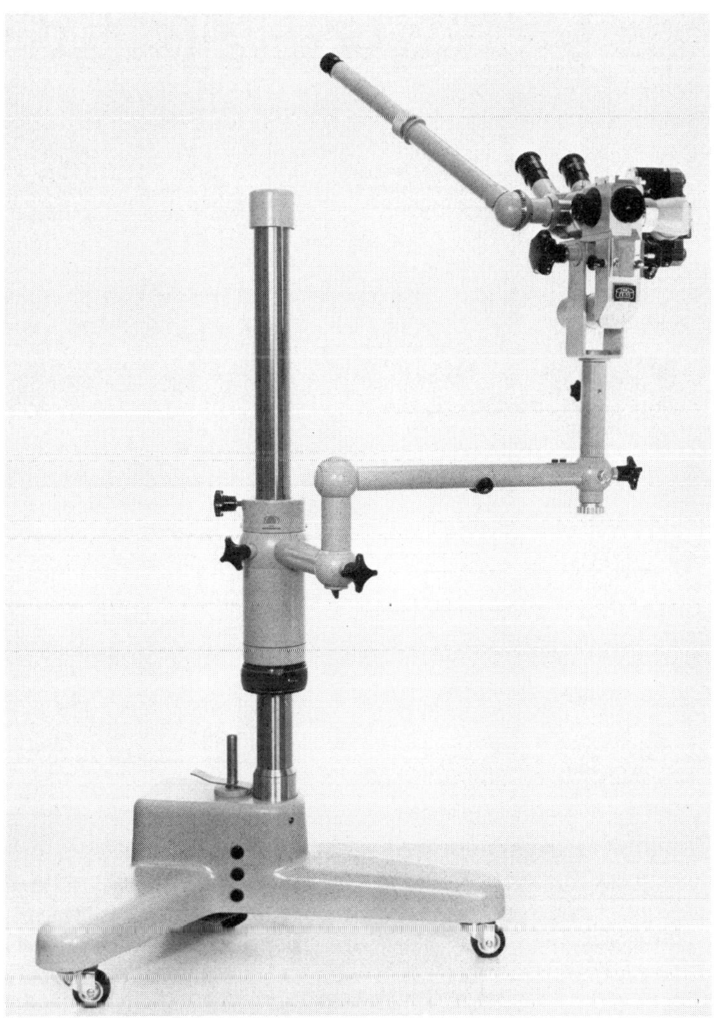

Figure 55. Zeiss colposcope 1 with camera and observation tube attached to colposcopic head. (Courtesy Carl Zeiss, Inc., New York.)

opens and closes the aperture diaphragm. The system is coupled with the exposure frequency (2 to 70 frames/sec). The film speed (10 to 400 ASA/11 to 27 DIN) is adjusted with a potentiometer. A cadmium-nickel battery serves as the power supply and for the control of all camera functions and for the diaphragm setting motor.

An extension cord and switch allow an assistant to operate the camera on command while the colposcopist focuses and carries out biopsy procedures.

Special eyepieces with an outline of the field being photographed are available in 10×, 12.5×, and 16×. With Super-8 film the object field recorded is rectangular, 4.2 × 5.7 mm. With a principal objective of 200 mm focal length, rectangles of 20 × 27 mm, 8 × 11 mm, and 3.2 × 4.4 mm are obtained with Galilean changer settings of 6, 16, and 40, respectively.

TELEVISION

For monochrome television, any commercial closed circuit television system may be used in which the camera has a standard C-mount. In order to limit excessive weight on the colposcope and retain its freedom of movement, small and lightweight television cameras are desirable. Since the picture size obtained in cameras of this type is slightly larger than that of 16 mm film, the f = 137 mm cine adapter is used (Fig. 56).

The addition of a lightweight color television camera has added a new dimension to the art of colpophotography. The authors have had experience with both Magnavox and Hitachi television transmission.

The Hitachi is a single tube color television camera using a 1 inch special vidicon with a built in frequency multiplex color filter as an image pick-up tube. The camera control unit has an external focus control which can be used to adjust the electrical focus of the image pick-up tube. When this control is rotated, the focus and color quality on the monitor screen vary. When this control is set at the optimal position, the red and blue components of the object are reproduced in best quality over the entire screen.

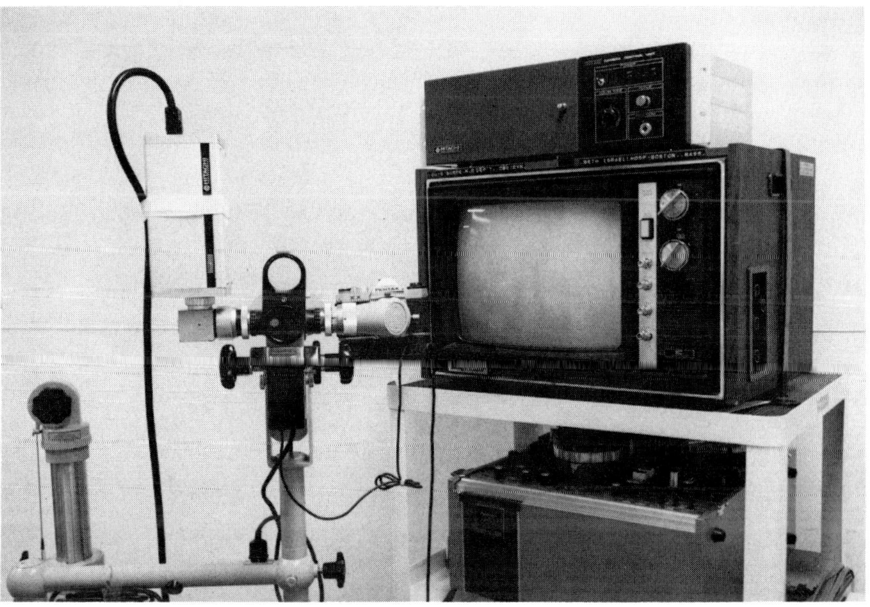

Figure 56. Television and videotape set-up with Zeiss colposcope 1. With this apparatus, patients are able to observe their own examinations which are also recorded on videotape.

Another external control provides adjustment of color tone. Clockwise rotation increases the red component and counterclockwise rotation enhances the blue component.

The Hitachi camera appears slightly more exact in resolution and reproduces somewhat finer colposcopic detail than the Magnavox counterpart. On the other hand, it is more sensitive to light changes and the diaphragm opening must be watched more carefully. With Galilean settings of 6, 10, and 16 a diaphragm opening of 15 is usually adequate; a setting of 25 requires a diaphragm opening of 11.

Television cameras have brightness control that is very sensitive to reflection and uneven lighting. Matte or Teflon specula should be used and the object areas evenly illuminated.

The following diagram shows the appropriate television connections for camera and viewer:

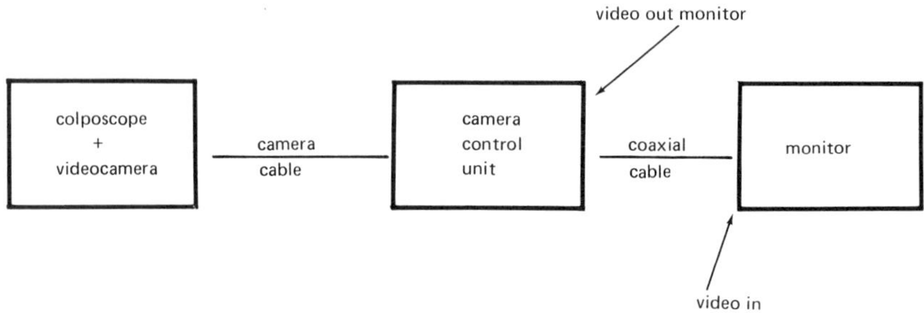

VIDEOTAPE RECORDERS

Television transmission of colposcopic examinations can be recorded on either reel or cassette forms of videotape recording. The authors have had experience with both the Sony and the Panasonic NV-3160 recorders. The latter permits one to edit the tapes. Both have facilities for recording or dubbing sound after the pictures have been taken.

The following diagram demonstrates connections required for television and videotape (VTR) recording:

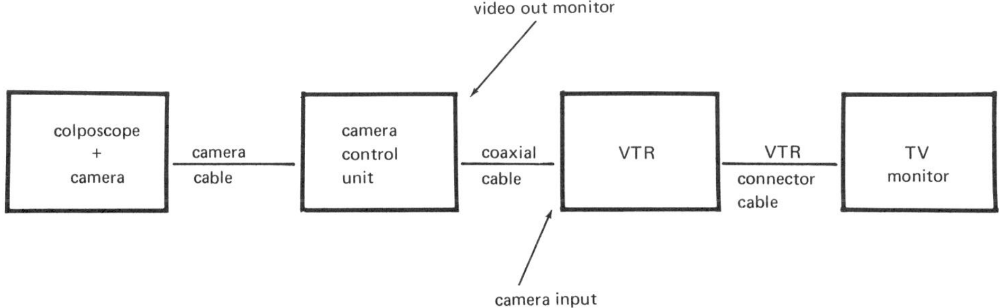

Additional monitors can be attached, especially for use at a distance from the room in which the colposcopic examination is being conducted. The following diagram is one method of setting up the monitors:

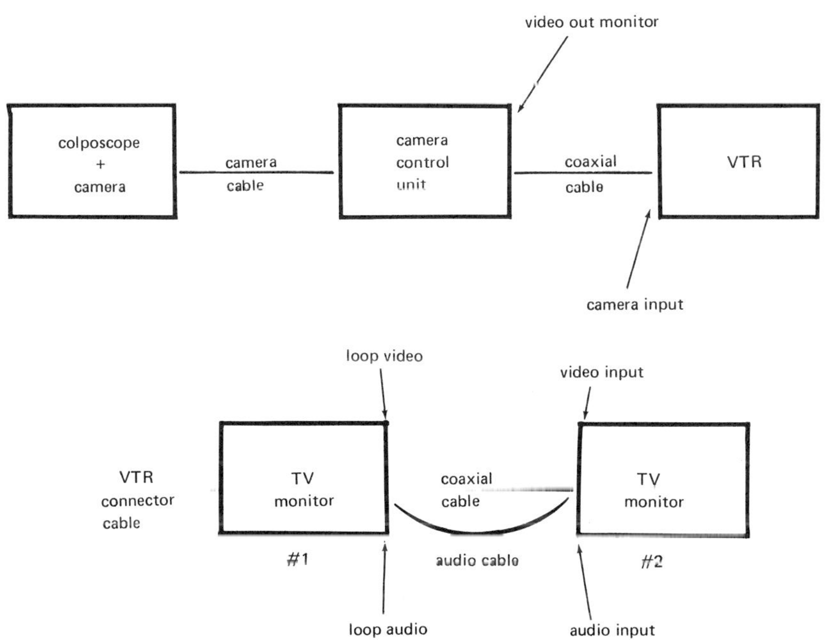

APPENDIX

MANUFACTURERS AND/OR DISTRIBUTORS OF COLPOSCOPES

1. Atlantex & Zieler Instrument Corp.
   55 Eastern Avenue
   Dedham, Massachusetts 02026

   (Distributor of Zeiss Colposcope and accessories.)

2. Applied Fiberoptics, Inc.
   46 River Street
   Southbridge, Massachusetts 01550

   (Manufacturer and distributor of Applied Fiberoptic Colposcope and accessories.)

3. Berkeley Bio-Engineering, Inc.
   600 McCormick Street
   San Leandro, California 94577

   403 Chestnut
   Union, New Jersey 07083

   (Manufacturer and distributor of Berkeley Stereo Colposcope and accessories.)

4. Cryomedics, Inc.
   500 Bostwick Avenue
   Bridgeport, Connecticut 06605

   (Manufacturer and distributor of KRY-med Colposcope and accessories.)

5. Dynatech Cryomedical Company
   90 Cambridge Street
   Burlington, Massachusetts 01803

   (Distributor of Jena Colposcope and accessories.)

6. Frigi-Scopes, Inc.
   A Frigitronics Company
   770 River Road
   Shelton, Connecticut 06484

   (Manufacturer and distributor of Frigi-Scopes Colposcope and accessories.)

7. Gynemed Inc.
   2458 Embarcadero Way
   Palo Alto, California 94303

   (Distributor of Leisegang, Zeiss, and D. F. Vasconcellos colposcopes and accessories.)

8. Gyne-Tech Instrument Corp.
   1111 Chestnut Street
   Burbank, California 91506

   (Distributor of Toitu Colposcope.)

9. Medical Specialties—Northeast, Inc.
   Danbury-Newtown Road
   Newtown, Connecticut 06470

   (Distributor of Toitu Colposcope.)

10. Carl Zeiss, Inc.
    Zeiss House

444 Fifth Ave.
New York, New York 10018

(Manufacturer and distributor of Zeiss colposcope and accessories.)

MANUFACTURERS AND DISTRIBUTORS OF BIOPSY FORCEPS AND EQUIPMENT

1. V. Mueller
   Division of American Hospital Supply Corp.
   6600 West Touhy Avenue
   Chicago, Illinois 60648

   (Tischler and Eppendorfer biopsy forceps)

2. Sparta Instrument Corporation
   305 Fairfield Avenue
   Fairfield, New Jersey 07006

   (Eppendorfer biopsy forceps)

3. Tuzik Instruments
   82 Chickatawbut Street
   Boston, Massachusetts 02122

4. All colposcope manufacturers and distributors previously listed.

MISCELLANEOUS EQUIPMENT

1. "Scopettes" (8 inch) may be obtained from:

   Fuller Laboratories, Inc.
   Eden Prairie, Minn. 55343

   (Stock #34-7021-8)

2. Styrofoam circles may be obtained from:

   Lipshaw Company
   7446 Central Avenue
   Detroit, Michigan 48210

BIBLIOGRAPHY

Antonioli, D. A., and Burke, L.: Vaginal adenosis: analysis of 325 biopsy specimens from 100 patients. Am. J. Clin. Pathol. 64:625, 1975.

Bajardi, F., Lang, W. R., de Maraes, A., et al.: Symposium, colposcopy of the irradiated cervix. Acta Cytol. 3:369, 1959.

Bechtold, E., and Reicher, N. B.: The relationship of trichomonas infestations to false diagnoses of squamous carcinoma of the cervix. Cancer 5:442, 1952.

Beller, F. K., and Khatamee, M.: Evaluation of punch biopsy of the cervix under direct colposcopic observation. Obstet. Gynecol. 28:622, 1966.

Bellina, J.: Gynecology and the laser. Contemp. Obstet. Gynecol. 4:24, 1974.

Bolten, K. A., and Jacques, W. E.: *Introduction to Colposcopy.* New York, Grune and Stratton, 1960.

Bolton, K. A.: Practical colposcopy in early cervical and vaginal cancer. Clin. Obstet. Gynecol. 10:808, 1967.

Bonfiglio, T. A., and Patten, S. F.: Histopathologic spectrum of benign proliferative and intraepithelial neoplastic reactions of the uterine cervix. J. Reprod. Med. 16:253, 1976.

Burke, L., and Antonioli, D.: Vaginal adenosis: factors influencing detection in a colposcopic evaluation. Obstet. Gynecol. 48:413, 1976.

Burke, L., Antonioli, D., Knapp, R. C., et al.: Vaginal adenosis: correlation of colposcopic and pathologic findings. Obstet. Gynecol. 44:257, 1974.

Cartier, Rene: Colposcopy, *in* Atlas D'Endoscopie Roussel. Les Laboratoires Roussel, Paris, 1974, chaps. 11-20.

Chanen, W., and Hollyock, V. E.: Colposcopy and the conservative management of cervical dysplasia and carcinoma in-situ. Obstet. Gynecol. 43:527, 1974.

Chanen, W., and Hollyock, V. E.: Colposcopy and electrocoagulation diathermy for cervical dysplasia and carcinoma in-situ. Obstet. Gynecol. 37:623, 1971.

Cope, I.: The colposcopic appearances with adenocarcinoma of the cervix. Aust. N.Z.J. Obstet. Gynaecol. 4:73, 1964.

Coppleson, M.: Colposcopy, cervical carcinoma in-situ and the gynecologist. Based on experience with the method in 200 cases of carcinoma in-situ. J. Obstet. Gynaecol. Br. Commonw. 71:854, 1964.

Coppleson, M.: The new colposcopic terminology. J. Reprod. Med. 16:214, 1976.

Coppleson, M., and Reid, B. L.: A colposcopic study of the cervix during pregnancy and in the puerperium. J. Obstet. Gynaecol. Br. Commonw. 73:575, 1966.

Coppleson, M., and Reid, B. L.: Origin of premalignant lesions of cervix uteri, *in* Taymor, M. L., and Green, T. H., Jr. (eds.): *Progress in Gynecology*, Vol. 6. Grune and Stratton, New York, 1975, pp. 517-539.

Coppleson, M., Pixley, E., and Reid, B.: *Colposcopy: A Scientific and Practical Approach to the Cervix in Health and Disease*. Charles C Thomas, Springfield, Ill., 1971.

Coppleson, M., and Reid, B. L.: *Preclinical Carcinoma of the Cervix Uteri: Its Origin, Nature and Management*. Pergamon, Oxford, 1967.

DePetrillo, A., Townsend, D. E., Morrow, C. P., et al.: Colposcopic evaluation of the abnormal Papnicolaou test in pregnancy. Am. J. Obstet. Gynecol. 121:441, 1975.

Dexeus, S., Carrera, J. M., and Coupez, F.: Colposcopy, *in* Friedman, E. A. (ed.): *Major Problems in Obstetrics and Gynecology*, Vol. 7. W. B. Saunders Co., Philadelphia, 1976.

Feldman, M. J., Kent, D. R., Linzey, E. M., et al.: The making of a colposcopist: a safe and sensible approach. J. Reprod. Med. 16:73, 1976.

Forsberg, J. G.: Cervicovaginal epithelium: its origin and development. Am. J. Obstet. Gynecol. 115:1025, 1973.

Forsberg, J. G.: Estrogen, vaginal cancer and vaginal development. Am. J. Obstet. Gynecol. 113:83, 1972.

Herbst, A. L., Kurman, R. J., and Scully, R. E.: Vaginal and cervical abnormalities after exposure to diethylstilbestrol in utero. Obstet. Gynecol. 40:287, 1972.

Herbst, A. L., Poskanzer, D. C., Robboy, S. J., et al.: Prenatal exposure to stilbestrol: a prospective comparison of exposed female offspring with unexposed controls. N. Engl. J. Med. 292:334, 1975.

Herbst, A. L., Scully, R. E., and Robboy, S. J.: Problems in the examination of the DES-exposed female. Obstet. Gynecol. 46:353, 1975.

Herbst, A. L., Ulfelder, H., and Poskanzer, D. C.: Adenocarcinoma of the vagina; association of maternal stilbestrol therapy with tumor appearance in young women. N. Engl. J. Med. 284:878, 1971.

Hill, E. C.: Preclinical cervical carcinoma, colposcopy and the "negative" smear. Am. J. Obstet. Gynecol. 95:308, 1966.

Hinselmann, H.: *Colposcopy* (with a section on colpophotography by A. Schmitt). Wuppertal-Elberfeld, Girardet, 1955.

Hinselmann, H.: Verbesserung der inspektions moglichkeit von vulva, vagina und portio. Munch. Med. Wochenschr. 77:1733, 1925.

Koller, O.: Colpophotography as an aid in the study of vulvar lesions. Acta Obstet. Gynecol. Scand. 45:88, 1966.

Kolstad, P.: The colposcopical diagnosis of dysplasia, carcinoma in-situ and early invasive cancer of the cervix. Acta.

Obstet. Gynecol. Scand. 43(Suppl. 7):105, 1965.
Kolstad, P.: The colposcopical picture of trichomonas vaginitis. Acta. Obstet. Gynecol. Scand. 43:388, 1964.
Kolstad, P., and Stafl, A.: *Atlas of Colposcopy*. University Park Press, Baltimore, 1972.
Krumholz, B. A., and Knapp, R. C.: Colposcopic selection of biopsy sites. Obstet. Gynecol. 39:22, 1972.
Kurman, R. J., and Scully, R. E.: The incidence and histogenesis of vaginal adenosis. Hum. Pathol. 5:265, 1974.
Lang, W. R.: Benign cervical erosion in non-pregnant women of childbearing age. Colposcopic study. Am. J. Obstet. Gynecol. 74:993, 1957.
Lang, W. R.: The respective roles of cytology and colposcopy in obstetric and gynecologic practice. J. Reprod. Med. 16:249, 1976.
Lang, W. R., and Ludmir, A.: A pathognomonic colposcopic sign of trichomonas vaginalis vaginitis. Acta. Cytol. 5:390, 1961.
Limburg, H.: Comparison between colposcopy and cytology in the diagnosis of early cervical carcinoma. Am. J. Obstet. Gynecol. 75:1298, 1958.
Littmann, G., Riedel, H., and Jakubowski, H.: Assistant's viewing tube and cine (television) adapter for Zeiss microscopes. Zeiss-Information 75, 1970.
Littmann, G., and Wittekindt, R.: Operating microscope with new photographic adapter and new secondary viewing tube. Zeiss-Information. 58:149, 1965.
Littmann, H., and Walz, W.: Colpophotography. Photographie Forschung. 5:2, 1955.
Mestwerdt, G., and Wespi, H. J.: *Atlas der Kolposkopie*, 4th ed. Gustav Fischer Verlag, Stuttgart, 1974.
Navratil, E., Burghardt, E., and Bajardi, F.: Simultaneous colposcopy and cytology used in screening for carcinoma of the cervix. Am. J. Obstet. Gynecol. 75:1292, 1958.
Nyberg, R., Tornberg, G., and Westin, B.: Colposcopy and Schiller's iodine test as an aid in the diagnosis of malignant and

premalignant lesions of the squamous epithelium of the cervix uteri. Acta Obstet. Gynecol. Scand. 39:540, 1960.

Odell, L. D.: The use of the colposcope in the detection and management of patients with early cervical neoplasia. J. Reprod. Med. 16:235, 1976.

Odell, L. D., Merrick, F. W., and Ortiz, R.: A comparison between negative, slightly atypical and suspicious cervical smears and colposcopic observations. Acta Cytol. 12:305, 1968.

Odell, L. D., Navratil, E., Richart, R. M., et al.: What is the place of colposcopy in modern gynecologic practice? Lying-In: J. Reprod. Med. 1:17, 1968.

Odell, L. D., and Savage, E. W.: Colposcopy, *in* Wynn, R. M. (ed.): *Obstetrics and Gynecology Annual 1974.* Appleton-Century-Crofts, New York, 1974, pp. 473-507.

Olson, A. W.: Colposcopic examination in a combined approach for early diagnosis and prevention of carcinoma of the cervix. Obstet. Gynecol. 15:372, 1960.

Ortiz, R., and Newton, M.: Colposcopy in the management of abnormal cervical smears in pregnancy. Am. J. Obstet. Gynecol. 109:46, 1971.

Pixley, E.: Basic morphology of the prepubertal and youthful cervix: topographic and histologic features. J. Reprod. Med. 16:221, 1976.

Plaut, A., and Dreyfuss, M. D.: Adenosis of vagina and its relation to primary adenocarcinoma of vagina. Surg. Gynecol. Obstet. 71:756, 1940.

Ruffolo, E. H., Foxworthy, D., and Fletcher, J. C.: Vaginal adenocarcinoma arising in vaginal adenosis. Am. J. Obstet. Gynecol. 111:167, 1971.

Sandberg, E. C., Danielson, R. W., and Prince, E.: Benign vaginal adenosis. Obstet. Gynecol. 30:93, 1967.

Savage, E.: Correlation of colposcopically directed biopsy and conization with histologic diagnosis of cervical lesions. J. Reprod. Med. 15:211, 1975.

Schellhas, H. F., Fidler, J. P., Rockwell, R. J., et al.: Resecting vulvar lesions with the CO_2 laser. Contemp. Obstet. Gynecol. 6:35, 1975.

Schmitt, A. W.: Practical application of colposcopy. J. Reprod. Med. 16:207, 1976.

Scott, J. W.: Colposcopy and colpomicroscopy, *in Davis' Gynecology and Obstetrics*. Vol. III, Chap. 18N. Harper & Row, Hagerstown, 1971.

Singer, A.: The uterine cervix from adolescence to the menopause. Br. J. Obstet. Gynecol. 82:81, 1975.

Sonek, M. G., Bibbo, M., and Wied, G. L.: Colposcopic findings in offspring of DES-treated mothers as related to onset of therapy. J. Reprod. Med. 16:65, 1976.

Stafl, A., and Mattingly, R. F.: Vaginal adenosis: a precancerous lesion? Am. J. Obstet. Gynecol. 120:666, 1974.

Stafl, A., Mattingly, R. F., Foley, D. V., et al.: Clinical diagnosis of vaginal adenosis. Obstet. Gynecol. 43:118, 1974.

Stafl, A., and Mattingly, R. F.: Colposcopic diagnosis of cervical neoplasia. Obstet. Gynecol. 41:168, 1973.

Thompson, B. H., Woodruff, J. R., and David, H. J.: Cytopathology, histopathology and colposcopy in the management of cervical neoplasia. Am. J. Obstet. Gynecol. 114:329, 1972.

Townsend, D. E.: Colposcopy, *in* Glass, R. H. (ed.): *Office Gynecology*. Williams & Wilkins, Baltimore, 1976, pp. 111-132.

Townsend, D. E.: Colposcopy: symposium. Contemp. Obstet. Gynecol. 6:66, 1975.

Trombetta, G. C.: Colposcopic evaluation of cervical neoplasia in pregnancy. J. Reprod. Med. 16:243, 1976.

Wilbanks, G. D., and Richart, R. M.: The puerperal cervix, injuries and healing. A colposcopic study. Am. J. Obstet. Gynecol. 97:1105, 1967.

Wilds, P. L.: Is colposcopy practical? Obstet. Gynecol. 20:645, 1962.

INDEX